Whole Motion

Whole Motion

Training Your Brain and Body for Optimal Health

Derek Beres

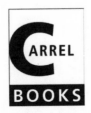

Carrel Books may be purchased in bulk at special discounts for sales promotion, corporate gifts, fund-raising, or educational purposes. Special editions can also be created to specifications. For details, contact the Special Sales Department, Carrel Books, 307 West 36th Street, 11th Floor, New York, NY 10018 or carrelbooks@skyhorsepublishing.com.

Carrel Books® is a registered trademark of Skyhorse Publishing, Inc.®, a Delaware corporation.

Visit our website at www.carrelbooks.com.

10 9 8 7 6 5 4 3 2 1

Library of Congress Cataloging-in-Publication Data is available on file.

Interior photos by Josh Nelson, unless otherwise noted.
Photo model credits: Callan Beres and Derek Beres, unless otherwise noted.

Cover design by Rain Saukas
Cover photo credit iStock

Print ISBN: 978-1-63144-072-4
Ebook ISBN: 978-1-63144-073-1

Printed in the United States of America

Contents

To my father, Ferenc, for kicking me into motion at an early age.
Thanks to him I've never stopped.

PART I
Setting the Stage

Chapter 1

An Introduction to Change

"The evolution of our unique brains was locked into the evolution of our wide range of movement. Mental and physical agility run on the same track."

—John J. Ratey and Richard Manning, *Go Wild*

THE ART OF MOVEMENT

Change, the old saying goes, is the only constant. But change itself is neutral unless we make it either positive or negative, resist or embrace it. We speak positively of being adaptable or resilient in the face of change, yet we often fear the inevitable rearrangements and reshaping of our lives, caught up in rituals and safeguards. While good habits that suspend distraction and make us productive are essential, overcommitting to routine can act as a barrier to the kinds of change that keep us flexible, growing, and truly strong.

This book is about motion, disruption, and regeneration, predicated on an understanding that exercise is as important for your brain as it is for your body. The exercise we do, and the journey of fitness I'll ask you to go on with me, is as much about training your mindset as it is about training your body. The rejuvenating effects

3

on your brain we'll discuss in these pages are every bit as important as the enhancing effects to your physique. Variety is not just the spice of life; it is also the key to true fitness. Learning to embrace variety and change—and the discipline to practice active regeneration, an essential pillar to our foundation—will give you greater control, pleasure, and strength, which positively affects your whole life, regardless of age. Why else would we work out? If change is the only constant, growth should be the only goal.

There are changes we have no say in: the loss of a friend or partner; a destructive house fire; learning you have cancer—that one certainly changed me. The real mark of self-control is how you deal with what you don't necessarily want or expect. Do you respond calmly or with fiery rage? How long does it take you to bounce back from adversity: minutes, hours, weeks? Are you able to let grudges go? These questions concern your health as much as how many burpees or pull-ups you can do. In fact, they directly affect how well you physically perform, in the gym, on the trail, and in life.

To understand how the tangible, physical reality of our bodies meshes with the interior, reflective landscape of our minds, consider the following. See if any of these mindsets describe you:

- Does yoga or meditation freak you out?
- Do you skip the stretch portion after a high-intensity class?
- Is your first response to a challenge to be anxious or stressed?
- Do you judge your performance against others?
- Is "ultra-marathon" an immediate turn-off? What about "5k jog"?
- Do you spend more time on the treadmill texting, reading, or chatting than focusing on your form, mechanics, and breathing?
- Is focusing hard for you?
- Is sweat the true marker of your workout?
- How about the "burn"?
- Do you use exercise to cheat at dinnertime?
- Do you obsess over the nutritional info on food labels?
- Is it hard for you to remember sequences even if you perform them regularly?
- Do you not show up if there's a substitute instructor?

If none of these describe your mindset, congratulations! These are but a few common patterns addressed in these pages, however. Your mindset toward health underlies how you relate to your body and mind, and no one has just one fitness mindset. In over a dozen years of teaching, I've noticed most students and clients seek to advance in some capacity. They're not just in maintenance mode. How they're progressing—working on handstand press-ups, training for a 100k trail race, spending more time in meditation and recovery—is an individual pursuit. What relates them is this relentless drive to grow.

And that involves changing things up. We often overlook the fact that we have the power to change every day. Your mindset helps determine whether or not you'll implement a new routine, if you'll stick with it, and if it's the type of change you really need. If anything in your movement vocabulary is lacking—flexibility, strength, better breathing capacity, the ability to focus for sustained periods of time—is it really impossible, or are you just not putting in the right amount of effort? Are you overtraining, or never even giving it a shot? Ask yourself how often you've started a sentence with, "I wish I could," "I really should," or "One day I hope to." If these statements resonate, this book will help you change that inner dialogue.

Sometimes we need an intervention. Disrupting habits is necessary for clarity of mind and body. If we're talking optimal health, being the best we can possibly be every day, we must discuss physical, mental, and emotional states. Yes, this book features cutting-edge research on fitness and exercise, but that's only one aspect of health. Your body does not move through the day lugging a disconnected brain. Everything works together, so you want everything in top shape.

The importance of integrating brain and body science is a hot topic. Since I began teaching at Equinox Fitness in 2004, I've observed a number of trends emerge. The most important is a growing dialogue between main studio fanatics—those who go hard in High Intensity Interval Training, who love metabolic conditioning, strength training, and Tabata, and who hit the trails and train for marathons regularly—and those entering the yoga studio for stretching, breathing, recovery, and meditation. Some need to get their heart rate up; others need to down-regulate more often. I've had numerous conversations with students about what they need to bring balance into their lives. I've watched some rise to the occasion. I've also listened to many talk about goals as a distant dream, apparitions with no basis in any reality they can imagine. Yet imagining is the first step in dreaming your goals forward.

You're now holding the result of such conversations. Change is not as hard as you think. Whether you need motivation to start a program or the patience to actively engage in regenerative practices such as yoga and meditation, it all begins with creating a proper mindset. Throughout these pages you'll be empowered with information necessary to accomplish just that. As you begin, it's important to note that this book is not presented as a cure-all because there is no singular program that works for everybody. There's no exact plan for any two people. What I hope to offer is a wide range of information and movements that can be tailored in creating a personal program in your pursuit of optimal health. As you begin the following exercise program, keep in mind that it's not necessary to perform them in the order listed. While the book is designed to flow as in a real exercise routine, you can always mix and match depending on what you need that day. The map is not always the territory, and so this book is designed for you to empower yourself as the designer.

START AT THE TOP

We assume that exercise makes us feel great because we're releasing stress, growing stronger, and becoming more flexible. While these are important markers, Harvard clinical professor John J. Ratey writes, "the real reason we feel so good when we get our blood pumping is that it makes the brain function at its best."[1] When we lift weights and run for miles we're stressing our bodies. The neurological response to these stressors makes us healthy. So don't think of stress as only a six-letter word. Soon I'll ask you to rethink your relationship to stress and its many different forms. Hopefully we'll figure out how to use the chemical reactions that create stress for our benefit while dissolving the unnecessary aspects of anxiety through active regeneration.

Let's face it: anxiety and tension are rampant in modern culture. I suffered crippling panic attacks for decades, including two that sent me to the emergency room and another that caused me to black out in a restaurant. Yet anxiety is also unavoidable, as it's part of our evolutionary heritage. Besides offering techniques to calm the cortisol rush, I'm also going to ask you to embrace certain elements of stress as part of developing a healthy relationship to your body and mind.

Another relationship we'll focus on is the one between your body and nervous system. Feeding your brain with the right movements, thoughts, and nutrition is an indispensable piece in this interlocking puzzle we call health. How we're acting in those twenty-three hours outside of the gym, track, or studio is as important as the hour we put into moving. A well-functioning brain is continually refreshed, which is why regeneration—rest, active recovery, and the ability to fine-tune thinking and resilience levels—is an integral part of well-being.

The slower side of fitness is often the hardest for people to grasp. For years I've watched students vigorously exercise in high-intensity classes and pedal with ungodly resistance in studio cycling. When the post-workout stretch arrives, they snatch their water bottles and run for the door. By engaging in this go-go-go mentality, they're also damaging their performance *during* class. They laugh it off by boasting that their "Type A" personality doesn't allow for stretching and breathing. Yet stillness is harder than movement. Thoughtful movement is more valuable than hard movement. Their excuse most likely reveals an inability to slow down, a skill that can be learned with time and patience. Before I began practicing yoga, I studied capoeira, a Brazilian martial art and dance form. One important lesson I learned during those six months, which has directly influenced all styles of movement I've practiced since, is that if you can do a movement slowly, speed will come. The opposite is not true, which has great implications on the load we place on our nervous system. Rest, thoughtful and deep relaxation, as well as proper sleep are all extremely important in lightening that load.

These two basic premises at the heart of this book—exercising for brain *and* body, and regeneration, which in biological terms involves cellular renewal, restoration, and growth—are not separate categories. You need to recover so you can give your all while working out in the gym and in life. By understanding how exercise affects your brain, you're educating yourself about the most important organ in your body. When you learn to treat it properly, you achieve optimal fitness. You gain mastery over your mind and movements.

Besides feeling more comfortable in your skin, you'll receive numerous cognitive benefits, including increased memory, more thoughtful decision-making, and dealing with your emotional reactivity better. That light and peace you find at the end of yoga is useless if five minutes later your senses are under assault from road rage. Likewise, strength gains from a kettlebell class don't accumulate if you never massage your fascia. Go ahead and ultra-size anything; just remember that your joints will pay the price without a little tender loving care.

We're soon going to explore an entire range of movements. In the Movement section, I'll discuss the brain-body connection in more detail. This will include a bit of evolutionary history and physiology to help you understand *why* you want to perform the exercises in this program. Understanding how our ancestors moved is important for recognizing how the human body was designed to function. Unfortunately many training methods we engage in today are due to a lack of diverse movements that our ancestors would perform on a daily basis. In our quest for perpetual comfort, we've lost something primary to our species. Harvard paleoanthropologist Daniel Lieberman calls these "mismatch diseases"—ways that our modern environment does not support our biological inheritance that in turn creates a spectrum of unique ailments. Many of the forthcoming exercises are in response to destructive patterns developed by culture. We often think evolution only moves forward for our betterment. Unfortunately, that's not how it works.

After we briefly review the brain-body connection, I'll share the latest research in five different exercise formats: Feldenkrais, high-intensity interval training (HIIT), resistance training, yoga, and meditation. From this section you'll be able to build a successful foundation for optimal physical health through a broad range of movement and levels of intensity and relaxation. How you construct your workout will depend on what you need more (and less) of in your movement regimen. I consider the sample routines a map, not the territory. How you navigate will be up to you.

In the following section, Mind, you'll use that knowledge to optimize your mental and emotional health. This includes chapters on developing focus to enter flow states, ways to disrupt your home environment (and clear out distractions), using music for optimal workouts, and important nutrition research for brain and body health. Remember, turning it up at the gym is not going to make much of an impact if you're turning it off when you leave. This might seem like a fitness book, but really, it's a lifestyle book.

More specifically, it's a movement book. My life is based on movement: moving bodies during yoga, studio cycling, and fitness classes; moving thoughts with words; moving hips and hearts as a DJ and music producer. My personal and professional life revolves around moving broadly, diversely, quickly, and slowly. Even slow movement, as we'll learn in the chapter on Feldenkrais, is still movement. Meditation, for example, is the intentional movement of thoughts, just as our imagination is the open-ended movement of ideas. Once you consider life a continuous pattern of thinking, moving, and feeling, you empower yourself to move in the direction of your choosing. The world might not always move in the same way, and so you'll learn skills to move through surprises and shocks as well. That's fitting, as the first step on our journey together involves disruption.

THE POWER OF DISRUPTION

We don't like being interrupted when we're focused on a task. Yet, when engaged in a mindless pursuit or a job we dislike, we welcome any novel break for a quick dopamine hit. Why else would everyone stare at their phones in line instead of engaging with one another? Or completely ignore the cashier because they want to know how many people liked their latest Instagram selfie? Talking to others is hard; gazing at your palm, simple. We intentionally disrupt our interactions all the time, leading to weaker social bonds, as well as strengthening our inability to pay attention to what's in front of us.

What we're concerned with is an intentional disruption of harmful movement patterns—and by movement I mean thinking as well. Neuroscientist Rodolfo Llinás believes thinking is a form of internalized movement.[2] He noticed that thinking fires motor neurons, the same pathways to actual movement. To test his theory, try to stop your thoughts and see how it goes. Even expert meditators recognize that thinking never ceases.

Rather than stopping our thoughts, we want to develop a thinking foundation that helps us achieve our highest good. We fall victim to habitual patterns of thinking just like we get stuck in movement routines: the same coffee each morning, the same route to work, the same thirty minutes on a treadmill. Repetitious exercise hypnotizes us with an illusion of growth; the same happens with thinking. The mountain we believe we're climbing is really a hamster wheel.

This can change. Even though psychologist William James first mentioned plasticity[3]—the idea that behavior can change throughout our lifetime—in the late nineteenth century, it was not until the 1970s that neuroscientists realized the adult brain is malleable. Until then, it was widely believed that once neuronal connections were set in early adulthood, that was that. Now we know we can change habitual patterns anytime, thanks to synaptic pruning. The more you move your body in a particular way, the more your brain map wires that pattern. To disrupt that pattern, you need to change the way you move. The same applies to your thinking and emotional life.

Moving differently, just like thinking differently, creates new neural pathways. For example, taking alternate routes to work is a wonderful way to strengthen your brain's hippocampus, the region implicated in spatial understanding and memory. The term "proprioception" refers to your understanding of spatial perception, how you move through space. The more you move the same way, the more that is the only way you know how to move. When you're stuck in such patterns—big or small—you become inflexible. The same trend holds true in religion, politics, sexuality, and pretty much every habit we can name.

Try this experiment. The next time you have to hammer a nail, use your left hand (if you're right-handed). Or (carefully) slice your vegetables with your non-dominant grip. Lately I've been cleaning my windshield with my left hand. I've also been prepping onions, garlic, and peppers with carefully orchestrated slices by my foreign fingers. Little changes make big differences, setting off a cascade of creative effects throughout the day. Upon changing one motion, your curiosity multiplies. You begin switching up other patterns.

Recently I watched a man practicing box jumps. Before each leap, he stepped back with his left foot. I suggested he try his right, which surprisingly challenged him. It also created a new movement pattern, as well as potentially balancing what could, over time, become chronic strain on one side of his body. Think about the imbalance in your right leg from handling all the foot action while driving, or the tension on the default hand with which you hold your phone.

I challenge my yoga classes like this all the time. Why do we always step forward with our right leg first? Ask many teachers and you'll likely receive an ambiguous response about the solar and lunar "sides" of your body. A more reasonable response is that this right side pattern developed out of convenience. It shouldn't surprise anyone that we favor that side, considering it is dominant in most people. As with many habitual patterns, we choose what's convenient and later invent the reason.

Optimal health is not convenient, however. Mediocrity is not an option if you're trying to fulfill your innate potential. Yet so many default to comfortable challenges in their fitness routines. You likely see the same people on the same machines and in the same classes, day after day, week after week. They've plateaued, no longer interested in growth. Sure, maintenance is better than not exercising. But you quickly become accustomed to patterns, even ones that were once overwhelming. You're receiving benefits but not achieving mastery. For that, you must disrupt your workout habits. The greatest effects of exercise are on your brain, and your brain craves variety. It wants new angles to explore, new mountains to ascend. So let's climb.

LEARNING WHOLE MOTION

My journey to optimal health has been—and remains—a lifelong process. I grew up in what appears to be two contradictory states: overweight and athletic. Due to poor dietary habits and the genetic luck of the draw, I carried around baby fat far longer than necessary. Yet throughout my youth I was active. I played every sport possible. My father encouraged it; he's still active. When not in uniform I was at the park shooting hoops, looking for friends to play wiffle ball, at the local street hockey spot, swimming laps as a lifeguard, on the golf course, or hackysacking in a circle. If there was a way to move, I wanted to try it.

The stretch between my freshman and sophomore years resulted in a big change. I entered high school about five feet, five inches tall; one year later I was nearly six feet. I kept growing in college, eventually hitting six-three. I didn't lose weight so much as I grew upward, but the new body felt good. During high school I played baseball and basketball while dabbling in hockey, tennis, volleyball, running, and golf. In college I kept up these routines, adding weight training and martial arts to my movement vocabulary.

Shortly after college I discovered Allan Wayne Work. This class is an exhilarating and informative combination of modern dance, ballet, yoga, and somatic conditioning. While attaining my degree in religion at Rutgers I studied yoga texts, but it was not until this class, held every Saturday morning in an NYU dance studio, that I began taking movement—especially slower, regenerative movement—seriously. I still remember the moment when my mentor, Brendan McCall, instructed us to perform a rotational hip movement while lying on the ground. I suddenly realized how little I knew about my body. I could barely extend my leg in the direction and at the angle he requested. I decided I was going to change that. I disrupted all my other workouts to set out on an exploration that is now two decades in the making.

Though training in martial arts (Tae Kwan Do and capoeira) had been difficult, yoga challenged me in new ways. Yoga was gaining in popularity in the nineties, though American cities and suburbs were not nearly as saturated as they are today. I was often the only man in class, which has fortunately changed; men appear to be more likely to focus on ultimately irrelevant goals, such as ripped abs or how much they can bench. There's nothing wrong with the desire to improve, but as Michol Dalcourt, inventor of my favorite fitness tool, VIPR, repeatedly emphasized during a workshop, there's a big difference between being fit and being healthy. After years of sports, weights, and cardio, I was learning the necessity of regeneration, through *pranayama* (breathing exercises), meditation, and deep postures. Yoga changed me from the inside out.

From there I kept exploring movement modalities with yoga as my foundation. When enrolling in yoga teacher training in 2003, I was employed as an editor at a world music magazine. I had been a full-time journalist since leaving college in 1997. Year by year I became increasingly fascinated with music from around the planet. I voraciously read about and traveled to as many countries as possible, learning what I could about their cultures—an early instance of introducing variety to my mental vocabulary. In fact, my love of various music and movement occurred simultaneously. It was also at this time that I began studying the neuroscience of music, to better understand why I love it so.

Studying your brain is in many ways the basis of Buddhism. One of the more famous observations is that when you meditate you become the observer observing the observed. Apply that to neuroscience: your brain studies how your brain operates. We might have different language for it, but yoga is similar, which is unsurprising given that Buddha practiced under two yoga masters before developing his own system.

While there are hundreds of styles of yoga today, they are all concerned with the search for the self. Since we now know that what we call the *self* results from neurochemical and environmental processes—our brain and body in constant conversation with its surroundings—it made sense to study the organ responsible for this process. While my research began with music, soon I was studying how movement affects my brain. Unsurprisingly, both music and movement have tremendous effects on our states of consciousness and physiology, a topic I explore in depth in Chapter 12.

All of this led to a fascination with neuroscience, music, and movement, a passion that served as the basis of a group fitness program I created for Equinox with my friend, Philip Steir, and our guide, Lashaun Dale. For three months Philip and I traveled around the country training yoga instructors how music and movement affect neurochemistry, and how to use both to create optimal class environments. For the next two years we wrote curriculum for dozens of instructors that were using this program as a platform for their classes. In many ways this book began with that program, inspiring me to study why a diverse range of movement affects our brain, as well as how our thinking and emotional patterns affect how we move.

While living in Brooklyn, I used to swim at the Park Slope YMCA. Above the pool were three words that defined the organization's philosophy: mind, body, spirit. This triune is meant to encompass the critical facets of being human. Rather than spirit, I consider emotions the essential third factor. What we refer to as *spiritual* usually involves grappling with complex emotional responses, as well as our relationship with our environment and culture. Regardless of terms, these three components are necessary for being healthy, productive humans. When we ail in one, the other two suffer. They can support or destroy one another. In the pages ahead, I hope to help you build the best possible support system.

This system is why I wrote this book. I'm not selling you a one-size-fits-all approach to health. It doesn't work. We all have different genetic, cultural, and environmental influences. Each of us needs to put in the work to better understand how to interact with our surroundings and deal with the constantly shifting fluctuations of our feelings and thoughts. Your brain and body are in constant conversation with everything around and inside of you. You only need to pay attention to hear the lessons and put in the time and effort to achieve mastery.

The dialogue between your brain and body invites you to be whole. Let's take that conversation to another level.

Chapter 2

Brain and Body

"It is your mind, rather than circumstances themselves, that determines the quality of your life. Your mind is the basis of everything you experience and of every contribution you make to the lives of others. Given this fact, it makes sense to train it."

—Sam Harris, *Waking Up*

OUR FIRST INSTINCT

We were born to move. Movement comes so naturally we rarely consider the complex symphony of physical and neurochemical processes that allow us to hurl our bodies through space. This is a good thing: we wouldn't travel far if we had to think about putting one leg in front of the other every time we take a step. Nature has programmed in us many unconscious processes so that we can focus our mental efforts on important issues. This phenomenon that we call "consciousness" affords us an ability to create technologies, imagine mythologies, and engage in self-reflection, all thanks to the partitioning of attention that cognition allows.

You can move even if you don't understand how. When you study the intricate orchestra playing between your brain and body, however, you can restructure your relationship to your body. Recognizing chronically poor movement patterns, for example, inspires you to learn better ones. Likewise, when you identify adverse nutritional choices you gain an ability to change your mind. The same holds true with intellectual nourishment, the media we consume. That's powerful.

In the pages ahead you'll be empowered with resources and information to make better decisions. Yet I'm not going to demand that you do this or that. No one-stop movement plan fits everybody (or even every body). My hope is that by providing you with the latest brain and body research you'll understand how to best design your own physical and mental fitness program. The sample workouts are examples of what I teach to my classes, a guideline to get you moving. From there, your personal creativity and integrity are the keys to success. The exercises are performed with your body weight so that you can do them anywhere. If you have a floor or a patch of grass, you're in business.

What matters is that you get moving. I don't discriminate. Advocates of various movement forms often claim theirs is best. I don't buy it. I'll try any workout. Don't misinterpret that; I love learning from masters of a discipline. All movement has an effect, and for the most part any movement is better than none. (Curling hand weights while on a studio bicycle? A little common sense is required.) Throughout these pages you're going to move as diversely as possible. You might try new things. You might slow down; you might speed up. Most importantly, you might have some fun.

The quest for movement begins in an ancient brain region that propels us forward. Neuroscientist Jaak Panksepp calls it the seeking system.[1] It began with our ancestors searching for food and shelter and has transformed into a host of other necessities and pastimes, such as the quest for beautiful music, the impetus to climb mountains, and riding along on epic adventures in novels. Inspired by those seeking their highest self, we stop at nothing to attain our own. Movement is one way to achieve this wonderful state of being. The neurochemical cocktail produced when we take care of ourselves is life-affirming and transformative.

As Taoists would say, let's focus on the journey and surrender any regard for the destination. In these pages I hope to let loose of the notion of the "perfect" or even "ideal" body. Being fit means feeling good inside of your skin, being comfortable with the person you are—and this is as much about your mental state as any physical feature. There is no perfect body type. But you can achieve an optimal state of health. In truth, it's quite simple. We've just set up so many obstacles that it can be hard to see.

After all, your fitness routines should be fun. In fact, "play" is my favorite word. You play at life all the time; your movement patterns should reflect this. Think of when you were young (or maybe recently?), rolling down hills and jumping up on curbs to test your balance. You might not consider such activities exercise, but they are. My favorite current exercise is trail running. Every moment offers a new landscape and different challenges for my feet, joints, and brain. While the uphill slog requires my lungs to work harder than ever, I often find myself skipping up on rocks and hopping over roots. When playing you're testing boundaries, learning what's possible. You pause your habitual movement patterns—work, car, table, bed—to test your will. You move outside of the box, eventually realizing there's only the box that you yourself built. Upon understanding this you build a more spacious playground in which to move about. We might all have certain restrictions due to genetics or injuries, but self-imposed boundaries are something we can do without.

Going to the gym to do this many reps or making sure to walk this many steps is the best way to destroy any sense of play. While some people are motivated by the tracking capabilities, the glorification of numbers creates unnecessary tension that, in a vicious feedback loop, causes an obsession over what is (or is not) being accomplished instead of enjoying the freedom of movement. That is the first mindset to disrupt, that you're working out for effect and not pleasure. If you're not enjoying movement, it's simply not worth it.

More disruptions are required, but I don't want to jump ahead. For the rest of this chapter, let's focus on the connection at the heart of this book: the intersection of your brain and body. We often consider fitness in terms of our body and psychology of our brain, but they are not separate. Never have been. Never will be.

Brain States

Understanding consciousness is a challenge for neuroscientists and researchers. We have many apt metaphors (and a number of silly ones) for the brain, in our attempts to describe how the brain works. The exact mechanisms underlying consciousness might not be discovered for some time, but metacognition—to know that we know—is in part what separates humans from other species. We have evolved an ability, in the words of philosopher Thomas Metzinger, to make "a reality appear *within itself*. It creates inwardness; the life process has become aware of itself."[2]

That inwardness does not result in only one mental state. Our brain actually exhibits two major modes. Numerous social and psychological ailments have arisen because humans can't differentiate between these two states, an especially pressing problem in our current age of distraction. Knowing when to be in one or the other is a critical piece in the overall picture of health.

The first is the default mode system, or mind wandering. We all daydream. In fact, the average person experiences two thousand daydreams every single day, each one lasting an average of fourteen seconds.[3] This tendency is not an aberration. It's what our brain does when left to its own devices. Spacing out and drifting off is important for our imagination and emotional health, if performed at the right times. Problems occur when we drift at the wrong times, such as when we text and drive.

The other mode is the central executive network, or focused control. This involves being so engrossed in a task, physically or mentally, that time seems to dissolve: getting lost in a great book or running ten miles in a flash. This mindset leads to flow states, which we'll discuss later. If you're concentrating on these words and how they relate to your life, you're in central executive mode. If you can't recall the first sentence in this paragraph, you've been drifting.

There are other differences between these modes. Humans can delay gratification, a rare trait in the animal kingdom. When in default mode we'll act in accordance with our mammalian cousins by seeking out a reward at that moment. While in executive mode, however, we realize holding off might just be a better option.[4] One danger of always responding to your phone is that it keeps you on constant alert, circumventing your ability to delay gratification, which in this case means not checking the moment the device dings. This results in long-term problems with attention and memory.

There is no "right" brain mode, though there are better times to be in one or the other. We're constantly switching between the two; both have practical applications. The challenge involves knowing when to be in one instead of the other. Mentally wandering while lying on the floor with your legs on a bolster after a hard day's work is a great usage of default mode. Texting your friend while at an intersection, not so much.

Differentiating between these two states is further confused due to an evolutionary oddity. Since at least the beginning of recorded time, and probably much longer, humans have believed that another entity—an energy, a soul—lives inside of their bodies in a phenomenon known as dualism. As we now know, that's simply not true.

MIND-BODY CONNECTION

Over the last four centuries, Cartesian philosophy has greatly impacted humanity's understanding of itself. French mathematician and scientist René Descartes is famous (or infamous) for his take on dualism, an idea that long precedes him but found a champion in his work. Simply put, dualism is the concept that our body and mind (or soul) are separate substances. (To be fair, Descartes was most interested in championing reason over emotions; dualism emerged as a consequence of his philosophy.)

Descartes did, in fact, evolve a groundbreaking idea that still holds weight. He believed the mind and body are uni-directional, a unique assumption during a time when many of his contemporaries thought the mind, an ethereal substance, controlled the earthly processes of the body, though not vice-versa. Descartes felt the body *could* influence the mind, though he still gave precedence to the mysterious mind itself. In modern terminology, he was a neocortex fan, the most recently evolved part of the mammalian cortex.

Alas, Descartes was misguided. What we call "mind" is a collection of neural processes, most immediately what we call consciousness. (It should be noted that consciousness is heavily influenced by unconscious processes as well.) The brain and body are in constant feedback. Considering the brain is *inside* of the body, it would be hard to fathom any other relationship. As the common slogan in neuroscience goes, "the mind is what the brain does."

Yet we are born dualists. Due to a range of chemical reactions and social conditioning, we enter this world feeling that a separate mind, or soul, exists independently of our body.[5] Consciousness, comprehending the environment and your place in it, is body dependent—no body, no mind. Without letting this become a religious argument, what should be recognized is that our thoughts greatly influence our body, just as what we do with our body affects our mind. Poor thinking often results in poor movement patterns; the opposite is also true. That's why optimal health involves fueling and moving your brain *and* body in the best possible ways. Humans have a habit of putting off what they believe is not within their control; dualistic thinking can serve as a buffer between idea and implementation. When you recognize all of your varied facets as one unified process, it's easier to make changes and fulfill ambitions.

Let's put this into context. Try this simple experiment that I've conducted for years in my classes. Sit comfortably for a minute or so. Close your eyes, simply to slow down whatever is happening around you; tune into how your body *feels*. Take slow, protracted breaths. When your mind has calmed, allow your shoulders to protrude forward and your chin to drop, as if you were hunching over a steering wheel or staring down at your phone. Notice the physical sensations corresponding with this action. Return to your starting position after a few breaths. Then take a few more breaths, attempting the opposite: draw your shoulder blades in and down, lift your sternum and chin slightly, and breathe fully. Observe the physical qualities associated with this simple alignment adjustment.

Hunched over syndrome is common. Sitting on chairs with ninety-degree angles—whoever dreamed up this anatomical monstrosity deserves a level in Dante's circles—for hours every day wreaks havoc on our body. Health professionals claim that sitting all day is as bad for your body as smoking cigarettes.[6] Unfortunately, a standing desk is not the antidote, as diversity of movement is more important than taking up one position for hours on end. A blend of standing and sitting is better. Personally, I take writing breaks every half hour to walk, stretch, or bother my cats. I also recently invested in a standing-sitting desk, so that every fifteen minutes I hit a switch and change positions.

Driving and texting are also implicated in this postural syndrome. Recall our experiment. Did you observe different sensations between the two postures? Could you tell that your breathing was stunted when rounded forward? Did your body feel lighter when lifting your sternum and chin? How you carry yourself is of great importance to your emotional outlook. It's the difference between shouldering the weight of the world and moving toward the light, two apt metaphors for very different ways you can move through the world.

The good news is that if you don't like how you move, if hunched over syndrome causes you to carry a burdensome load, you can change that. Simple shifts have the potential to result in profound changes. We sometimes overlook the subtle, mundane patterns of everyday life to focus on big-picture items. Unfortunately, this mindset begins in the wrong place. To better understand, let's peek at the process of how we remember anything and everything, as all our patterns start with memories.

TOTAL RECALL

You've probably heard the term "muscle memory." Learn a movement pattern, and that'll be how you move, for better or worse. Muscle memory falls under one of two major categories of remembering. As a *procedural* memory, muscle memory is a form of motor learning, in which repetition creates habitual patterns of movement—walking, running, even sitting and posture. We become accustomed to moving in a particular way. Our brain solidifies these patterns.

Changing how you move can be overwhelming, as if you're suddenly asked to acquire a new body. In some ways, you are.

To understand why variety and regeneration are so important to our health, we need to briefly explore how memory works. There is declarative memory, further broken down into episodic memory, which allows us to gaze back into the past and recollect events, and semantic memory, the storage of facts. Interestingly, the neural regions responsible for episodic memory are also what allow us to predict the future. Rarely will anyone guess future events without being influenced by their past because our brains use the same system to comprehend time.

By contrast, *implicit* memory is unconscious. These are learned procedures: riding a bike, tying your shoelaces, getting to work every morning. A lot of cognitive resources are devoted to learning a task, but when unconscious it becomes part of our implicit memory system. This skill set allows us to focus on other tasks without, for example, relearning how to put one foot in front of the other each time we walk—unless we're retraining our gait to change our muscle memory, of course. Then we make conscious what we one day hope to become unconscious. This is how we learn, unlearn, and relearn.

We often think of episodic memories as being stored in our brain the same way files are saved on a computer: put something in and there it rests until we open it again. Our brains are not hardware, however. It's seductive to consider our skull's interior as elegantly designed as our laptop. It's just not true.

When something happens, you observe it. But it's not just you at that very moment—it's the *you* that includes your catalog of biases, perceptions, and beliefs. Pure memory is a misnomer (although a miniscule percentage of the population does have "perfect memory"), which is why episodic memory is malleable. For example, I might be trailing a car as it smashes into the truck in front of it. I observe a sudden slamming on the brakes, skidding, impact. What I do not see, but what someone standing on the sidewalk does, is that the guilty driver was staring at his phone. I might learn that later on, which would likely alter my memory of the event. In fact, much of what we remember changes as new information becomes available.

Then we believe we witnessed something that we never did. I'm now certain the driver's head was down, oblivious to the road in front of him. I might even recall a green glow shining upward from his lap. My personal narrative has changed dramatically without *my* even being aware of it. Perspective is everything, but time shifts perspective. New details emerge in the future; my past has changed.

We don't recall any event unblemished. Instead, we reconstruct each memory. During the process we're constantly altering the past. If you've ever wondered why you get stuck mulling over an event—a break-up, the death of a loved one, losing a big game—it's because each time you recall it you're rewiring the circuitry of that memory. The inner vision persists, often growing stronger as time separates you from it. As your present changes so does your history.

As poet Marie Howe puts it, "Memory is a poet, not an historian."[7] Memories are processed in our brain's hippocampus, a word derived from the Greek term for "seahorse" due to its physical resemblance. Located in our cerebral cortex, this region is responsible for short- and long-term memory as well as spatial navigation. It is also implicated in memory loss and disorientation during Alzheimer's disease as well as other ailments of decline.

As it turns out, movement greatly decreases the onset of such diseases that involve cognitive decline. In an aging world with a growing population, 15 percent of those over the age of seventy-one suffer from dementia; an additional 22 percent are afflicted with mild cognitive impairment.[8] This results in a $109 billion annual bill in America. According to researchers at the Mayo Clinic, the most important benefit of seniors moving their bodies is "improved neuroplasticity and neurogenesis." The growth of BDNF (more on this below) and insulin-like growth factor, IGF-1, results in "significantly larger hippocampal volume."[9] Their ability to remember improved when moving their bodies more often. Yet often we don't realize this until we're dealing with the problem in real time. This is advice we can heed now in order to stave off future concerns.

Adding variety into your movement patterns is also helpful. As with thinking patterns, how you move through space changes the structure of your brain. Muscle memory might better be termed motor memory. Remember Llinás's observation that thoughts fire motor neurons. Just because certain motor memories no longer require conscious effort does not mean neurochemical processes are not occurring every time you move. This is why quality of movement is so important. Everything you do impacts your brain and memory system. Build bad patterns and you suffer unnecessarily. Build better ones and you feel the freedom of an uninhibited body and mind.

I often witness new students showing up to yoga with a trademark slouch. Simply getting them to elongate their spine takes tremendous effort, often requiring a bolster or yoga block to sit on. They have to learn an entire new skill set that will hopefully become unconscious over time. With enough patience and effort, their spine aligns with their shoulders above their hips. Their entire demeanor changes as they become softer, stronger, and more perceptive of their environment. What took Herculean struggle becomes effortless. Nothing inspires me like watching people recognize progress right before their eyes. Learning better memories changes your future. But this is only half the story. The other half cannot be seen, but it sure can be felt.

MORE TO BELIEVING THAN SEEING

You've heard the expression "I'll believe it when I see it." We are visual creatures. When discussing health, it doesn't help when magazine covers constantly promote ripped abs and toned arms. Remember, being fit does not necessarily mean being healthy. I'm not dissuading you from seeking aesthetic results, but this emphasis on bodily features does a great disservice to what health actually means.

In many ways, health begins inside. Sure, there's the motivation and desire to become stronger, more limber, more in shape. There's also chemistry. Brain-derived neurotrophic factor (BDNF) is a protein that acts on our central and peripheral nervous systems. Produced by the ventromedial hypothalamus, BDNF helps our brain make and differentiate new neurons and synapses, the latter being the channel that allows a neuron to pass a signal to another neuron. BDNF supports higher thinking and motor control, showing another link between thinking and movement. As it directly affects the hippocampus, BDNF is critical in long-term memory formation as well as movement patterns. Certain exercises help grow BDNF, which also plays a role in neurogenesis, the birthing of new neurons. Basically, exercise helps our brain sprout new neurons while making more durable connections between existing ones. Both are necessary for sustained health.

To return to computers, our brain *is* like a hard drive in one sense: researchers believe memory is "a collection of information fragments dispersed throughout the brain."[10] (Hard drives disperse files into fragments, recollected when recalled. They just don't recall what has been saved since, unless the file is corrupted.) The hippocampus is the way station that collects and assembles these disparate pieces of information. As mentioned earlier, memories do not return in perfect order. Research has shown that one of the most prominent neural regions that BDNF appears in is the hippocampus. The more you exercise, the more it shows up. Not only does this help you remember more and better, it helps your rate of learning. The more complex movements you attempt, the more branches of this dendritic tree sprout. (Dendrites are the far-reaching projections of the neuron; under a microscope they mimic a tree.)

Movement is a language, with each pattern being one tongue. The more languages you speak, the more people with whom you can communicate. The more people you talk to, the less likely you're going to fall victim to unnecessary biases against others, and the more fun you're going to have engaging with a wider array of friends. This is better for you as well as society as a whole. Variety of friendships is healthy. Think of your brain as a vast social network. Every time you touch the furthest reaches you expand your knowledge exponentially. How we move outside is reflected by how we move inside.

Diversifying movements also has a social component. In gyms and studios you work out with varied groups of people. At Equinox many members exercise in three studios—main, studio cycling, and yoga—yet each room features distinct communities. Boutique studios are especially popular for assembling tight-knit tribes. Now think of your brain as a community. Runners are going to get the wonderful benefits of consistent cardiovascular exercise and endurance training. Adding yoga offers you an ideal flexibility and regenerative application to your repertoire. Throw in kettlebells, resistance training, dance—you see where this is headed. Not only will your body become stronger and more flexible, you'll constantly increase your brain's ability to form new connections. Your neural tree grows branches that apply to other aspects of life. You remember better, you learn better, and you *feel* better.

By taking responsibility for your health, you're increasing the likelihood that you'll live a long and healthy life. Mindset is an important component of this. Having a positive view of aging has shown to increase one's life span by eight years.[11] By feeling good physically and mentally, you're more likely to enjoy growing older than someone in chronic pain. Variety, the saying goes, is the spice of life. This particular spice is an essential ingredient to the endogenous cocktail your brain and body produces every single day of your life.

We are all born movers. Slowing down our movements does not come easily for many, however. To accomplish this you need to observe the subtler aspects of movement. This is where regeneration comes into play. Our movement journey begins and ends with mindful, regenerative practices, tracing back to the earliest stages of movement and ending with higher-order cognitive practices. Along the way your heart rate will go up, you'll become stronger and more pliant, and your brain will be flooded with the proteins and hormones that your body and brain crave, including BDNF, oxytocin, and dopamine. Before we roll and jump and meditate, however, let's start with the most basic movement of all: regeneration.

Chapter 3

The Regeneration Prescription

"Survival of the population, survival of the individual, and survival of the cellular structures that make up said individual all depend on the delicate balance of forces within the body."

—Katy Bowman, *Alignment Matters*

EDITING YOUR NARRATIVE

As an animal you're wired for arousal. Your brain is on constant alert for threats. Your ancestors had to be aware of what's around the corner, if that approaching stranger can be trusted, if that berry is edible. This genetic blueprint is encoded in you. While important historically, modern humans have exploited this alert system by focusing our attention on relatively benign problems. This underlying tension leads to a host of chronic problems—compromised immune functioning, gastrointestinal distress, poor sleeping patterns, and obesity, just to name a few—which is why recovery plays a critical role in optimal health.

Absolute stillness is impossible. But you can slow down your nervous system, which then allows you to attain a sense of mastery over your thoughts, feelings, and movements. Regeneration unlocks this important door. To wrap your head around why this matters, let's discuss movement once more.

We touched upon how the human brain uses the same system for remembering the past and portending the future. To navigate your environment, you're constantly predicting what occurs next. Movement is a form of prediction. How heavy is that package? Did that driver just slam on her brakes? Which way do I need to bend over to pick my child up? How is my posture while typing this book? What seems commonplace requires loads of unconscious (and sometimes conscious) biomechanical processing. Even when motor patterns are unconscious your brain is constantly predicting.

Now factor in a nervous system sensitive to stressors. In the absence of real danger we often invent it. How many times have you mentally written narratives that turn out false? Does your perception of yourself differ from what others tell you? Do you question yourself even though you know what you're doing? This is true for many of us. Yet it's not life creating this mindset; it's our brain's love for storytelling. If such tales live inside of your head, they're in your nervous system.

Sometimes you're the writer of your story. Sometimes you're the editor. Developing a healthy relationship to our bodies and brains requires both good writing and editing.

NOTHING TO WORRY ABOUT

Your nervous system is divided into two parts: the central nervous system (CNS), which includes your brain and spinal cord, and the peripheral nervous system (PNS), which deals with nerves that connect every part of your body to the CNS. While the CNS is the CEO, it is nothing without the efforts of PNS branches. If one worker is injured, the entire system is disrupted. The economic disparity between wealthy executives and underpaid staffers in modern society would never occur in our body. The entire system would shut down. We are interdependent beings in our interior design.

There are three components of the PNS (somatic, autonomic, and enteric), but for our purposes let's focus on the autonomic, as it is the most relevant to your regeneration experience. This system is further divided into sympathetic and parasympathetic. Dutch psychiatrist Bessel van der Kolk refers to the sympathetic as the accelerator and the parasympathetic as the brake to our body's energy resources.[1] The sympathetic system triggers the familiar fight-flight-freeze (FFF) mechanism. It's named sympathetic because it works *with* your emotions. When activated, blood rushes to your muscles, thanks to adrenal glands pumping adrenaline. When an unseen branch snaps in the woods, this system keeps you on high alert. Unfortunately, it is frequently unnecessarily activated. Many people live as if they're only hitting the gas and never braking, which is quite damaging over time.

For example, pretend you have your "spot" in your favorite yoga class. You always arrive twenty minutes early to ensure that your mat is placed in the correct position. One day an accident causes excruciating traffic. You pull into the studio with two minutes to spare. Your spot is taken. During the entire class you can't let the sequence of events go. You could have left home earlier. Why did that accident have to happen today? Who is that person in my spot?

This scenario is no invention. I've seen it happen. I've heard students yell at others trying to squeeze in near the start of class. This is an ultimately futile exploitation of their nervous system. There is no actual danger; nothing is *wrong*. You were not in the accident; you made it to class on time. You simply have to adapt to practicing in a different part of the room. And some people cannot—though they can, if they reorient their nervous system's response mechanisms.

This includes reorienting your beliefs about stress. While chronic anxiety is destructive, health psychologist Kelly McGonigal argues that creating a healthy mindset around stress is important. No response or emotion is inherently good or bad. What matters is the motivational direction. For example, anger is a powerful social tool that can result in policy changes on a governmental level or it can remain bundled up with no channel to express it. McGonigal points out that the more stressed a nation's citizens are, the higher that country's GDP and life expectancy—despite how counterintuitive that sounds.[2] Having a negative mindset around stress certainly creates problems, as in using "I'm so stressed" or "This is stressing me out" as a default response. Yet the hormonal charge of stressful situations is exhilarating, creative, and productive. As she writes, "Stress can create a state of concentrated attention, one that gives you access to more information about your physical environment."[3]

Motivational direction is important in every form of stimulation: stress, fear, joy, anger, contemplation. As we are always interacting with our environment, creating a proper mindset is essential. Of course, tragic and damaging experiences, such as rape and war, make it difficult to move forward. Dr. Bessel van der Kolk has written extensively about the ways that humans damage their nervous systems, especially in regards to trauma. Quoting his teacher, Elvin Semrad: "The greatest sources of our suffering are the lies we tell ourselves."[4] Such as, I need to be in *that* spot in order to practice yoga. That's an example of a benign, invented suffering. Even more challenging mindsets from traumatic experiences can be confronted and reoriented, however, provided that we slow our nervous systems down.

That's why you want to spend more time in parasympathetic mode. This system takes control when you're relaxing. The term means "against emotions," meaning you're working *against* FFF mode. PNS also aids in digestion and wound healing. The release of acetylcholine slows your heart rate, calms your breathing, and relaxes your muscles. When you drop into this state of relaxed sensation and open awareness, healing begins. This is the system we will activate later in this chapter.

CONTINUOUS DIALOGUE

The conversation between your body and brain never ceases. While it's possible to think yourself down from overstimulation, your autonomic system is insidious—it often operates outside of conscious control. The ANS sends signals to smooth muscles, glands, and cardiac muscle. When the sympathetic system enters FFF mode, your body mobilizes its energetic resources. In the short term—look out, a bear!—it plays a critical role in survival. Over time, as anxiety becomes chronic and motivationally damaging, your body remains on constant alert. This is a growing cultural problem. One study found that Americans collectively miss 321 million days of work every year due to anxiety and depression, costing the nation's economy $50 billion.[5]

Your sympathetic system never sleeps. This security system is necessary in case credible threats appear. Picture a skyscraper, which sways in the wind a number of feet in every direction. If it didn't, the structure would be too brittle and inevitably collapse. Too much sway and it crumbles as well. It is designed to be stable enough to withstand the elements, as is your body. In humans this balancing act is called homeostasis. In order to maintain it, your sympathetic system remains on. In a society that's always plugged in, however, we need to spend more time activating our PNS so that recovery and regeneration can occur.

Examples of homeostasis include maintaining a livable body temperature as well as proper blood acid and alkaline levels. When everything is working properly you feel good. No body part screams for attention. But this balancing act is precarious. While humans are hearty animals, it doesn't require much to take the entire network offline. A proper balance of movement, nutrition, and thinking patterns ensures well-being. Unfortunately, many situations—driving, sitting at a desk, sugar addiction, deluges of information on social media, chronic work syndrome—throw us off-balance.

So we need to look beyond homeostasis. While important, a more appealing mechanism is at play: hormesis. When receiving a vaccination, your doctor injects a low-level dose of a toxin into your bloodstream to strengthen your immune system. In fitness terms, hormesis is infecting your body to not only maintain balance, but to grow stronger. For example, when lifting weights you're purposefully creating inflammation and stress in your muscles. As long as you're not overtraining, you'll grow in size and strength. The temporary injury is beneficial.

Likewise, such an effect is possible with cardiovascular exercise. This can be specifically applied to anxiety. I spent much of my life in FFF mode. My first anxiety attack hospitalized me at age sixteen, then another a dozen years later. In fact, I've experienced hundreds of panic attacks. While a number of techniques have helped me conquer this condition, including the meditation and breathing exercises in this book, as well as seriously investigating my nutritional choices, a more aggressive trick helped me down from attacks. As it is called fight-*flight*-freeze, I decided to fly. Whenever an attack approached, I hopped on a treadmill or went outside and ran. After ten minutes the attack was gone. I co-opted an evolutionary trait to my advantage. I also grew stronger in the process. What I didn't know was that I was releasing the exact protein, BDNF, necessary for optimal health. This protein happens to be the star of regeneration.

Take a Load Off

Fear and anxiety are among the most prevalent psychiatric disorders in America, affecting 20 percent of the population.[6] Neuroscientist Joseph Ledoux argues that we have not inherited fear from our animal ancestors, but rather we've "inherited from them the capacity to detect and respond to danger."[7] Through a non-conscious alert system our anxieties commence, often appearing in seemingly unrelated circumstances: you're mad the barista took too long, but really, you're stressed about the extra work your boss dumped on you right before the weekend.

The environment you live in also plays an essential role. One study found that children living in a New York City apartment building whose windows face a subway track fare worse in reading comprehension than children on the quieter side.[8] The constant stressors of street noise negatively affect their nervous systems, which leads to all sorts of problems, from learning impairment to heart attacks.[9] Studies show that living near an airport has detrimental effects on health. Place matters.

Complete silence does not appear to be the answer, however. An "optimal amount" of noise, around seventy decibels, has been shown to "make your fingers more sensitive to sensations, improve your ability to see contrast, and even correct your posture (by enhancing 'proprioceptive,' or positioning, signals)."[10]

How to come to terms with our modern predicament? We often say we need more space, more quiet, more vacations—two weeks offered by most American companies is a joke among developed nations—but as Kelly McGonigal reports, "People are happier when they are busier, even when forced to take on more than they would choose."[11] Being attentive and, yes, busy are two ways to give our life meaning. Shifting your mindset to both invite stress as a motivational tool while remaining un-stressed about stress means we need to tap into the relaxed sense of focus that occurs when we're operating in our brain's executive function mode. This is where regeneration comes into play.

Regeneration is a key aspect in nature. Ever witness a forest after a fire? Ecosystems regenerate. So do bacteria. Most animal life regenerates. Fish and salamanders regrow limbs; humans do the same with their skin and liver. There are many examples of regeneration, but for our purposes we're looking at neuroregeneration, our ability to grow, rebuild, and repair nervous tissues, cells, and cell products. This occurs in the central and peripheral nervous systems, dependent upon the feedback of both brain and body.

Focusing on exactly what we're doing while in recovery mode aids this process of growth and healing. Tuning into our inner processes allows us to enter parasympathetic mode, leaving us refreshed, revitalized, and less stressed (in a good way). As a result, we think more clearly and make better decisions about our lifestyle, exercise, and nutrition. Our memory even becomes stronger and longer lasting.

Let's look at an example in everyday life. Think of your route between home and work. Do you notice the streets? How about the cars, or the people in those cars? Or do you aimlessly steer unaware of the signs you pass every day? Do you arrive at your destination with no awareness of how you got there, pulling into the parking lot as if on autopilot? Sadly, this is often the case.

Alfred Hitchcock famously stated that drama is life with the boring parts taken out. If you're paying attention there are no boring parts, which is why I focus on transitions in my classes: how you get from one posture or movement to the next. Every time you practice, an opportunity for growth and playful exploration exists. Whenever you sit to meditate, stretch, or breathe, take a moment to learn something new about yourself. Trail running affords me a rare hour or two to be by myself in nature with only the thoughts circulating in my head. Many ideas for this book and other works arise during these morning hours. Such revelations begin by noticing the subtle aspects of your environment while avoiding going on autopilot.

Whenever you move, especially when you move in different ways, BDNF floods your entire brain. The rush of novelty needs to be tempered by a cultivation of patience. This is the balance between hormesis and homeostasis: push your boundaries and then reflect on the new landscape. Push again; relax again.

For the rest of this chapter we'll explore my three favorite techniques for regeneration: myofascial release, breathing, and sensory meditation. All three offer access to parasympathetic mode. Before we explore these techniques, let's set the stage.

TIME TO RELAX

I suggest practicing regenerative techniques as often as you work out. It might not be for as long, but consistency is key. You can cycle through these and other techniques throughout the week. On workout days practice in the evening, just not right before bedtime. Since these exercises put you in parasympathetic mode, they will prepare you for sleep. But you don't want to be half-asleep when starting. Focus is needed.

I also recommend dedicating a space in your home for this work. I prefer my living room, near the balcony. Sometimes I perform these exercises in the bedroom, but since that space is dedicated to sleeping, a subconscious association exists. Having a regenerative space sets the tone. This also helps create a healing mindset in which to approach this work.

Our first exercise is a form of myofascial self-massage. Understanding the role of fascia is one of the great advancements in therapeutic massage and the movement arts over the last two decades. The term comes from a Latin word meaning "band," and it is exactly that: a band of connective tissue that acts as a "second skin" underneath your skin. Primarily composed of collagen, fascia stabilizes, encloses, and separates muscles and organs. When it gets tight or becomes otherwise compromised due to poor movement and posture habits, the entire system suffers. Jill Miller, creator of the popular regenerative yoga program, Yoga Tune Up™, calls fascia the "ubiquitous living seam system in your body that threads your tissues to one another."[12]

There are three forms of connective tissue in your body:

1. Hard tissues.
2. Soft tissues.
3. Fluid tissues.

Hard tissues include bone, cartilage, and periosteum, which surrounds bone. Soft tissues include tendons, ligaments, and fascia, while fluid tissues are blood and lymph. They are all composed of the same cellular components. Where each tissue is located and what it supports determines the firmness and composition. Miller writes that connective tissues play two major roles in your body: connection and protection. Depending on where it is, fascia is essential to both.

One of my favorite images from Taoism (and Bruce Lee) is to "flow like water." This is not merely a metaphor. Your body is mostly composed of this hydrogen-oxygen cocktail; fascia is water's storehouse. Think of a hike in which you encounter a stream generously flowing from its peak. There's a rhythm, a seemingly determined pace according to slope and environment. Now picture a dam formed from a fallen tree or a collection of rocks. A pool forms; the water no longer flows, struggling to trickle past the barrier. Due to poor postural and movement patterns, many of us suffer such dams: tight, condensed fascia that allows no flow. We're looking for fluidity and ease of movement. Addressing fascia is essential to accomplishing this.

One reason fascia is a relatively new science in therapy is because of its complexity. In an age of medical specialism, the role of this second skin has taken researchers time to understand. For example, many years ago my left shoulder locked up. My range of motion was compromised; a general ache forced my shoulder head forward. I visited my massage therapist, Loretta Young, who was an early student of anatomy trains. She spent twenty minutes working the fascia behind my right knee. When she was done there was no more left shoulder impingement.

As an instructor that sees hundreds of students and clients every week, I am often asked for advice regarding injuries. I never diagnose, as my area of expertise is not in medicine. I do have a catalog of movement variations they can apply, but my first reply is always to see their doctor. I usually follow this up, if applicable, by telling them to visit a good massage therapist that specializes in myofascial release.

Miller defines myofascia when she writes, "There is no muscle that does not have fascia winding its way throughout every layer of its cells and fascias and surrounding its whole structure."[13] You can understand why this is such an important system to address. We need our tissues in good working order. We want our entire body to flow like water. As my therapist loves saying, "Your issues are in your tissues." Fixing your tissues not only addresses your second skin, it also helps you regulate your emotional response to life's challenges. Chronic pain affects how you perceive and act in the world. Pain is a powerful motivational factor. Likewise, when you feel good, you're less likely to react in poor taste to life's circumstances.

In the following pages, I present the exercises that will help with regeneration. Please remember that all exercises in this program are demonstrated at wholemotion.com. For the first stage of recovery and regeneration, let's roll.

The Program: Regeneration
Exercise #1: Roll with It

While you can (and should) roll every part of your body, we'll focus on two areas that generally hold tension: your upper back and piriformis. There are a variety of tools available to assist you, though I'm partial to Yoga Tune Up™ balls. A tennis ball works as well.

Some therapists suggest harder objects, such as racquetballs or lacrosse balls. I find these too abrasive. You want to coax your fascia and muscles. You don't want to assault them.

It's important to remember that while there might be a small amount of pain, especially if you have trigger points, these exercises should not be torturous. I understand the desire to feel like a lot of work is happening. In terms of regeneration, less is often more. You're aiming to relax and heal your body; you don't want to approach these techniques as you would a HIIT class. The mindset is different, which is to be expected, as this is a holistic program.

This is the only exercise in this book requiring a prop. I've added it only because fascia release is essential for regeneration.

Let's begin with your upper back.

1. Lie down on the floor on your back in the space you've designated to healing. If it is hardwood you might want to put down a blanket, unless you're accustomed to that surface.
2. Slide one ball on each side of your spine under your upper trapezius muscles. You might have to play around to find the right spot; somewhere around the inner corners of your scapulae usually does the trick.
3. Walk your feet in so that you can touch your heels with your fingertips. Bridge your hips to the ceiling, allowing the weight of your body to roll on top of the balls. Close your eyes and take ten deep breaths, focusing on long exhales.

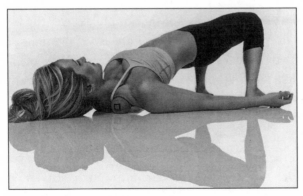

Photo by Samantha Jacoby

Photo model credit: Trina Altman

4. After ten breaths lightly roll along the grain of your muscles, shearing your skin atop the balls. Allow the balls to roll to the top of your trapezius muscles all the way down to your mid-back. When you find a tight spot, breathe deeply, lifting your hips to different heights to create more or less tension.

5. After five minutes of exploration, holding for ten breaths in various spots, lower your hips and slide the balls from underneath your back.

Now for your piriformis muscle, located in the gluteal region. It is a lateral rotator muscle that many people overlook when stretching and strengthening. Its tightness can cause lower back pain and a loss of flexibility in your hips. This is especially important, as piriformis syndrome, which occurs when the piriformis irritates the sciatic nerve, leads to sciatica. I suffered from this condition as a teenager after breaking my femur. Fortunately yoga, massage, and myofascial release helped me overcome it.

1. Lie on your back and place one ball under each buttock muscle, a few inches below your sacrum. With your knees bent, gently lift your hips to slide the balls under and feel the tight spot. From my experiences, it won't be hard to find.

2. Once in place, allow the weight of your body to sink over the balls. Take ten deep breaths.

3. Bringing the soles of your feet together, allow your knees to fall in opposing directions toward the ground. When you've reached the end range of motion, relax over the balls and take ten deep breaths. If your hips are especially tight you can slide two yoga blocks or pillows under the outside of each knee for support. Don't raise your knees too high. You want the weight of your legs to allow the balls to do their work.

4. Once you've become acclimated to the tension, slowly open and close your legs, bringing your knees toward one another and then opening them back up again. Slowly repeat ten times before drawing your knees into your chest and moving the balls away.

Exercise #2: PNS Breathing Technique

The word "spirit" comes from the Latin *spiritus*, "breath." Breathing taps into our emotional body. Learning how to breathe well has the potential to shift your outlook on life. It eases you, comforts you, and makes your skin fit more comfortably.

In the 1960s American physician and neuroscientist Paul D. MacLean proposed the "triune brain model," which has become the standard when discussing the architecture of the human brain. The three aspects are:

1. Reptilian complex.
2. Paleomammalian complex (limbic system).
3. Neomammalian complex (neocortex).

While it is easy to generalize how our brain is composed by claiming each "part" specializes in something distinct—emotion, memory, cognition, and so on—it is better to look at this model comprehensively: each region affects and influences others. We would not be rational animals without emotion. That said, the reptilian brain refers to your thrust for survival, your reactionary phase, your emotional response system. We *feel* before we think, regardless of how logical we are—an emotion is how we mentally translate a physical sensation. As you know, it is quite easy to be swayed by emotion. The key to working with emotional reactivity resides in your breathing.

Take a deep breath. Probably one of the most common responses to stress and anger ever uttered. But first, a caveat: *exhale deeply.* Your inhalation is important—when stressed it tends to be short and choppy—but a long exhalation causes your vagus nerve to send a signal to your brain to kick into parasympathetic mode.

I recommend trying the following exercise seated, though it is possible to practice while lying down. This might take a little getting used to. When people start elongating their breath it feels like swimming underwater. Go slowly; there is no rush. If you tend toward anxiety, remember that you're trying to work with it, not deny its existence. This mindset helps if you feel suffocated. Your body breathes without conscious direction anyway, so there is nothing to fear. Within a few minutes you'll be able to stretch your breath comfortably. Be diligent and patient with yourself.

1. Find a comfortable seat, on the ground or in a chair (or lying down, if neither of these is comfortable). Make sure your shoulders are directly above your hips. This alignment ensures that your vestibular system, your body's balancing mechanism, is doing the least amount of work.
2. Close your eyes. Removing visual stimulation helps you focus on breathing.
3. Begin with a deep breath through your nose followed by a long, sighing exhale from your mouth. I always perform two or three of these before any breathing exercise. That alone brings a sense of calm to my mind and body.
4. Inhale through your nose for a count of four, exhale through your nose for a count of eight. Counting gives your mind something to focus on. Over time you might not need numbers, but for the first minute or two it ensures your exhales are longer than your inhales. You might only accomplish a four-to-four ratio. That's fine. See if you can make it four-to-five, and so on.
5. Enjoy! Notice the sensations associated with slow, thoughtful breathing. Aim for at least ten rounds. Your body will most likely become more relaxed.

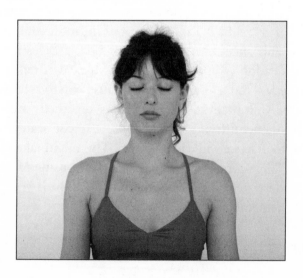

6. When you've finished ten rounds, sit for another minute or two with your eyes closed, letting your lungs breathe automatically. Notice the sensations associated with this exercise. Then recognize that parasympathetic mode is always only a minute or two away from almost any situation. This knowledge helped me deal with anxiety disorder. Being aware that an antidote to FFF mode is so close has kept me from spiraling into panic on a number of occasions.

Exercise #3: Sensory Awareness Meditation

The philosopher Alan Watts found it funny that we scrunch our forehead while weighing a decision. Why would we tighten our facial muscles, an act that restricts blood flow and signals tension, when what we're seeking is a calm, parasympathetic flow of information? We often combat tension with more tension, which obviously never works.

For this third exercise you're going to calm your nervous system through a sensory awareness body scan. This is a restorative way of bringing focus to various body parts so you can relax them.

Lie down in your healing space, on a blanket if you want a little softness underneath you. Remember, while this exercise is very relaxing, it's not meant to put you to sleep—though if you do it's not a big deal. Sleep is relaxing as well! If your lower back or legs ache, place a few pillows or yoga bolster under your knees so that they're passively bent. The gentle incline between your knees and abdomen further promotes parasympathetic stimulation.

1. Lying on the ground, notice the sensations in your feet and toes. Take a few moments focusing on each foot, observing how each feels. Then relax it. You might even flex and extend your toes a few times before letting them settle.
2. Move up to your calves. Spend a few moments focused there, then to the back of your knees, up your legs, and to your pelvis. After this first scan is done, take a few breaths, noticing both of your legs, from the pelvis down, completely relaxed.
3. Move your awareness to your hands next; begin with your fingertips. As with your feet, you might make fists and open them

a few times before letting them relax on the ground with your palms up.

4. Trace a line up your forearms, to your elbows, and up your arms to your shoulders, taking a few moments on each region. When you get to your shoulders, take a few deep breaths and allow them to soften. From here you'll work down to your abdomen. Spend a few moments there before taking deep breaths throughout your entire body, allowing everything from your neck down to melt into the floor.

5. Begin facial relaxation by moving your jaw and tongue around. Puff out and relax your cheeks. Keeping your eyes closed, squint and soften your eyelids. Once you've traced your face from bottom to top, flutter your lips. Imagine your brain resting in the back of your skull. Allow your head to be as soft as the rest of your body. Remain here for at least ten minutes, observing the sensations of your entire body. Ambient music is a great aid for this full body scan.

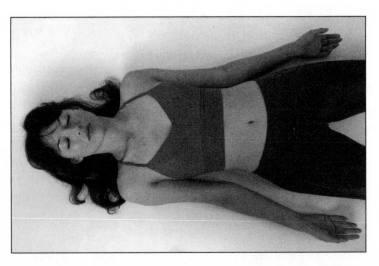

Everything functions better when you're relaxed and in less pain. The above techniques help calm your nervous system and put you in a state of receptive awareness and physical ease. This is only half of fitness—an essential and sometimes undervalued half. Movement is equally critical for the success of your health. So now, let's move.

PART II
Movement

Chapter 4

Learning to Crawl

"We shall do better to direct our will power to improving our ability so that in the end our actions will be carried out easily and with understanding."

—Moshé Feldenkrais, *Awareness Through Movement*

IN THE BEGINNING

It begins with a fire inside.

Earth formed in a similar manner as other planets: attracted to a star, in this case the sun. Debris of dust and rock circled this sun for eons, positioned at just the perfect distance to ride out billions of years of instability to eventually produce life. Over time, star stuff congealed and hardened. Thanks to a proliferation of carbon—the fourth most abundant element in the universe, the second most in the human body—the violent, chaotic orchestrations of matter heated and cooled, shouldering the brunt of asteroid impacts, which helped to form a dense shell over an unstable gang of isotopes. The fire inside of our planet raged, tempered by a crust molded through countless millennia of chance and proximity.

We were, in essence, born of movement.

If our planet had landed just a degree closer to the sun, life as we know it would never have occurred. Rather than speculate over what didn't happen, let's focus on how we came to be. This is no aside: our bodies are constructed from the same primordial soup that birthed everything. The chemistry is amazing and precarious. Minor variations in our bodies create substantial problems. The same holds true in our environment. Optimizing our chemistry is the best we can do in what remains a rather unstable existence.

While life requires a complex orchestra of elements, carbon is especially important. Carbon atoms link together and bind with other atoms, informing the structure of DNA. Besides silicon, no other element is as versatile and necessary. It helped the universe expand and created the structures that we stare at in the night sky. Carbon infiltrated this planet on the back of meteorites and comets, molding cosmic dust into what became our planet. Carbon combined with water and nitrogen, among other elements, to conceive the world we know today.

Not that animal life was immediately forthcoming. Atmosphere 1.0 didn't support oxygen breathers, steeped as it was with carbon dioxide and carbon monoxide, as well as suffocating levels of cyanide and phosphorus. There was a process of cooling, heating, and cooling again, before finally a balance was struck. While a diverse list of ingredients was present, no cook mastered the recipe. To this day there is no model of what life *should* be. Rather, life is what it is. We do our best to survive and, at this relatively peaceful planetary junction, thrive.

Thank cellular life for all that we have, what paleontologist Richard Fortey calls "a mass of chemical reactions surrounded by a skin."[1] To continue our analogy, I'll borrow from the Indian craft of Ayurveda: the digestive fires inside of our bellies nourish and sustain us in a similar manner that the explosive core of our planet sustains life. Our skin, like the earth's crust, is a container for chemistry. And it took quite some time to achieve. Some 3.5 billion years ago, the first cells emerged. Like a child with a set of LEGOs, life began building block by block, step by misstep by step.

Prokaryotes were first. The name for these single-celled organisms is derived from Greek, meaning "before kernel." These were late winter seeds soon to bloom. Bacteria comprise one type of prokaryote. The other is Archaea, which live in salt lakes, hot springs, soil, and skin. Prokaryotes reproduce asexually, predominantly through a form of regeneration called binary fission: a single entity splits into two parts. Along this evolutionary fission pathway a serendipitous divergence occurred. Sexual reproduction appeared to the pleasure of animals ever since. Eukaryotic cells—"eu" means "good," showing our appreciation for this evolutionary upgrade—allowed multicellular life to commence. As philosopher Daniel Dennett notes, "We are eukaryotes, and so are sharks, birds, trees, mushrooms, insects, worms, and all the other plants and animals, all direct descendants of the original eukaryotic cell."[2]

At the risk of reminding you of your high school biology teacher, let's note what's important: cellular reproduction requires movement. Through movement, primeval cells colluded, split, and united to form, at a proto-snail's pace, everything that exists on this planet. This movement had but one goal: reproduction. Repeat; start again. Cellular life was set into motion. It has not slowed since.

I'm going to skip over four billion years of animal evolution, from multicellular organisms through spineless seafarers, invertebrates, and vertebrates. And voila! We get to the nervous system, a beast that knows no pause. In order to move through space, you have to be aware that you're moving through space. Enter this complex and fascinating system nature programmed into animals to help us process everything tactile and sensational.

When you hear the term "neuroscience," you most likely picture a brain. Yet the field is actually devoted to the nervous system in its entirety, which comprises the brain and spinal column. The system as a whole is the true brain behind movement, and its individual parts are interdependent aspects of everything that you are. From external sensation and internal monitoring arises every conscious and subconscious activity your body needs to live. This extends to our environment, as we are in constant dialogue not only with ourselves, but everything around us. Fitness and ecology are longtime bedfellows, for the health of our planet and the health of our bodies are inseparable.

Everything interacts and responds to its environment. Even single-celled organisms detect and move away from threats—that's how they survived in the first place. They're also drawn to beneficial stimuli, just like humans are. But we're not one giant cell; every one of our thirty-seven trillion cells partakes in this endless dance of attraction and repulsion. The overseer of this dense network, your brain, is equipped with its own defense system to ensure fitness. Unlike single-celled organisms, human cellular power is multiplied when united, like a group of collaborating superheroes. Your nervous system incessantly monitors, sends out, and receives information from all of your organs and muscles, as well as the exterior world. Move away from that. Get over there, stat.

Of course, sometimes your nervous system becomes overloaded with stimulation—an expectable response in an increasingly technologized and easily distracted society. But we are not the same animals as just a few centuries ago; our ancestors moved much differently. Free from the chores of hunting and gathering, both of which by necessity involve movement, the extent of modern physicality often includes only thumbs and fingers, combined with any number of short trips to and from a vehicle. While this trend toward pacifism creates plenty of work for massage therapists and psychiatrists, as well as fueling an obnoxiously lucrative pharmaceutical industry, one of the greatest threats we face today is missing an email or not replying to a text within five minutes. Nature instilled in us an important threat detection system that we've short-circuited. To our advantage—to the point of this book—we can rewire it. We may have undone nature's long work, but evolution never moves in only one direction. How you want to move forward is completely up to you.

Changing your mind, like changing your body, takes work. For most mortals, change produces anxiety. The human nervous system, evolved to detect threats, is overworked by the incessant cartwheels of imagination. While Kelly McGonigal's work in mindsets regarding stress is important, let's face it: most fears are self-created. American workers who suffer from anxiety disorder take off twenty-five days every year due to stress, costing our economy an estimated $50 billion.[3] When the motivational direction of stress is chronic worrying and distress, the result is mentally crippling and emotionally exhausting. Anxiety is implicated in rising rates of obesity, depression, chronic inflammation, sleep troubles, and much more. To address fitness today forces us to confront how we relate to stress.

Neuroscientist Joseph Ledoux specializes in anxiety. The basis of this volatile condition, rooted in our FFF mechanism, is not so much existential stress as it is a necessary response to danger. Our fears exploit a system designed for more pressing concerns. As Ledoux explains, "The evolutionary function of this ancient capacity is not to generate emotions like fear or anxiety, but simply to help ensure that the organism's life continues beyond the present."[4]

Anxiety is especially pertinent to health thanks to the overwhelming number of people suffering such disorders, as well as the financial and social impact. This includes financial incentives for doctors to keep patients on anti-anxiety medication, in some cases over-prescribing them. I'm a case study myself. Once dependent on Xanax, it's been almost two years since my need for Xanax. While I never lean on anecdotal evidence alone, I'm confident the research and techniques that follow have the potential to help others.

We began this chapter discussing the evolutionary roots of movement. Anxiety creates movement in our physiology and psychology, and is therefore possible to control. Though one of the markers of anxiety is feeling disempowered, history tells a different story. Evolved from the *Australopithecus* genus of apes roughly 2.5 million years ago in East Africa, our ambitious forebears mated with and decimated populations of at least six other species of *Homo*.[5] Through an exploration of increasingly vast territories, armed with the gift of bipedalism and a prefrontal cortex that helped to create the complex communication system we call language, humans are equipped with the most intricate nervous system on the planet. Somewhere between one hundred billion and one trillion neuronal connections exist inside each of our heads. The sheer processing power of your brain is tremendous. Not bad for an animal whose origins reside in a single cell! The trick is getting your nervous system in top working order, to either eliminate or work with the stresses of existence. In order to start this process, you need to slow things down.

EXPLORING CENTIMETERS

Movement is easy. Stillness is the real challenge. To understand the relationship between your brain and the rest of your body, to refine the threat detection responses of your nervous system, slowing things down is necessary. By doing so, you're able to think and move with more confidence and ease, creating a stronger and suppler relationship with yourself and your environment. To accomplish focused control over your thoughts and movement you'll need to make the smallest possible articulations of your joints and muscles, which is a therapeutic modality in itself.

This is what Moshé Feldenkrais realized after tearing his meniscus and severely damaging knee ligaments while playing soccer. Born in what is now Ukraine in 1904, he spent a sizable portion of his life escaping prosecution for being Jewish. At fourteen he walked from Belarus to Palestine, picking up two hundred people along the way.

After Arabs attacked Jewish villages and his cousin was killed, Feldenkrais taught himself self-defense without the use of a weapon. This led to instructing others. One particular attack by knife-wielding Arabs left many Jews dead. Feldenkrais developed an intricate blocking technique to combat this social fury. Yet his students never mastered it; they could not resist the urge to block their faces or turn away. Watching students respond to a technique he thought foolproof was essential to the development of his system. From that day he no longer countered the instinctual responses of the nervous system. Instead he learned to work *with* it. This led him to study jujitsu and judo, both of which use an opponent's force against them. A lifelong learner, Feldenkrais eventually earned a PhD in physics while paying his way from teaching judo.

Feldenkrais went on to cofound a judo club in France even as his knee deteriorated. While he recognized that his knee problems were not psychosomatic, two things struck him as odd. First, his knee was worse on some days than others. Second, the pain was greater when he was mentally stressed. By chance he fell and injured his good leg. When he woke after a deep sleep, he was shocked to find that he stood perfectly well on his chronically injured leg. Your nervous system, as it turns out, will not learn new information when a region of your body is in pain.[6] The pain in Feldenkrais's newly injured leg superseded his chronic pain. This revelation taught him to restructure his nervous system. As psychiatrist Norman Doidge writes, "The acute trauma to Feldenkrais's 'good leg' led his brain to inhibit the motor cortex brain maps for that leg to protect it from further injury should he move. But when one side of the brain is inhibited, often the other takes over its functions."[7] Feldenkrais realized torn ligaments were not the only responsible agents. By retraining his brain to react to the motor responses, he altered his knee's condition. That meant he had to change his habitual movement patterns. The Feldenkrais Method was born.

I took my first Feldenkrais workshop in 2006. The focus of the entire two-hour class was getting up from the floor. At thirty-one I didn't see this as any great challenge, though in my classes I'd witnessed a number of people struggle with this endeavor. In fact, researchers in Brazil developed a "sitting-rising" test. They found that the more points of contact you make to get up off the ground, the more likely you're going to die sooner than people with no issue standing up.[8] Not only did I find Feldenkrais's techniques for this seemingly simplistic task valuable, my entire body felt incredible after the workshop was over. It is extremely meditative, thanks to a slow focus on minimal movements.

In 1972, Feldenkrais wrote, "When we refer to movement, we mean, in fact, the impulses of the nervous system that activate the muscles, which cannot function without impulses to direct them."[9] He knew that his postural habits hindered progress in rehabilitating his knee. He decided to remove antigravity muscles from the picture by lying down. From there he began an exacting investigation of tiny articulations, moving his leg hundreds of times in fractions of inches. He developed a holistic approach to his body thanks to an understanding that the somatic and psychic domains are not separate but interconnected and interdependent: there is no thought without movement and no movement void of thought. Treating any physical condition and refining habitual patterns require a tremendous amount of effort. Paradoxically, this sometimes means moving in the smallest possible manner, spending hours exploring centimeters.

This notion of miniscule movement flies in the face of fitness in a culture of Spartan races, extreme endurance challenges, CrossFit, and ultramarathons. Remember, Feldenkrais is a healing modality. Run a hundred miles in two days and recovery is essential. Run a mile and you still need to recover. Feldenkrais offers important insight into the nature of the brain-body relationship: After spending a half-hour relaxing one knee, he was able to accomplish the same on the other knee in just two minutes. This is thanks to priming: exposure to one stimulus prepares you for another. Once one side of your brain is ready to receive information, the information flows faster across the divide.

Feldenkrais also recognized that every thought corresponds with a change in musculature. In order for our brain to learn better patterns in thinking and movement, we need to slow our movements down. Feldenkrais knew from judo that "effortless action" is the way to defeat an opponent. This is no easy chore. It requires contemplation and education working in conjunction with easefulness and patience. Feldenkrais understood that real strength comes from relaxation; no valuable learning occurs when strained. There's an image from yoga that highlights this idea. One translation of the relaxing *balasana* (child's pose) is "strength posture."

It's important to note that Feldenkrais was also hip to a theory that would not be proven for a half-century after his knee injury: our brain can change itself. Obvious now, a contentious debate about the nature of our mind-stuff had raged for millennia. To this day, some believe that certain patterns of being are part of their genetic stock and therefore unchangeable. That's a shame, because such a belief is resoundingly false.

TAKE A CHILL

When the prolific psychologist William James proposed the idea of plasticity in his 1890 classic, *The Principles of Psychology*, his belief that neural patterns were not fixed was widely ignored. Even though vast transformations had for millennia been promised in the world's religious traditions (James's other field of study), psychologists clung to the notion that adults were unable to alter cortical maps. It took eighty years for science to catch up.

Part of the problem involved too much stargazing. The idea of localizationism infiltrated psychology for centuries. The astronomer Galileo Galilei is credited with coining the term. Spending his days staring into what he considered a "cosmic clock," he believed bodies were mechanistic cogs in the machinery of the universe. As with people today using computer analogies to describe the brain, Galileo believed the cosmos was a well-oiled machine, not a living, breathing organism susceptible to physics and evolution. His philosophy covered macro to micro: the hardwired brain is a collection of parts, just as the stars are. If one part is broken, it's unfixable. Physicians accepted this inevitability as a faulty design to be endured rather than tested. It took four centuries for science to destroy this theory.

Yet an ascetic monk named Siddhartha Gautama had tuned into the brain's changing states two thousand years earlier. The Buddha's Four Noble Truths, which gave rise to the Eightfold Noble Path, is essentially a prototype of neuroplasticity: there is suffering in this world; suffering happens because our perception is faulty; you can change your perception and therefore be liberated. While Buddha might not have discussed cortical maps, he was onto something important.

The term "neuroplasticity" is now common in the marketplace of ideas. There are two types of plasticity: synaptic, which involves how neurons connect with each other and is dependent upon usage, and non-synaptic, referencing changes within individual neurons. While the latter interacts with synaptic plasticity, it is considered separate. We're going to focus on synaptic plasticity.

It's easy to stare back at history smugly. With practices like trepanation (boring holes into the skull) common, understanding the electrical interplay of neurons was impossible. It was not until non-invasive technologies like functional magnetic resonance imaging (fMRI) afforded researchers an opportunity to investigate brains without directly affecting their patterns. We'd long known certain brain regions affect movement, sight, and speech, thanks to research on trauma and disease. With fMRI we gained the ability to look at the how those maps communicate across networks of neurons. The brain was no longer understood as a collection of parts but as an organic whole. This is important because it underlies this entire book: optimal health is impossible if you believe the seemingly disparate parts of life to be unrelated. That's why we're training them as one.

This is what Feldenrkais recognized during those many hours on his back subtly manipulating muscles and ligaments around his injured knee. The doctor who told him there was a 50 percent chance meniscal surgery would be useless did not understand the connection between cartilaginous tissue and the brain. Sadly, doctors today still overlook this. Seven hundred thousand arthroscopic knee surgeries are performed in the United States each year, a $4 billion industry[10]—I'm included in that figure, having had mine scoped in 2015 after a basketball injury. Not everyone benefits from this surgery. Personally, my pain has been greatly reduced, though no thanks to the post-operative machinery at UCLA. I was left to my own devices with little input from the operating team in terms of physical rehabilitation or somatic counseling. I attribute my healing process to movements inspired by Feldenkrais.

In fact, much of Feldenkrais's work is relegated to rehabilitation. While this wonderful modality has impacted countless people, most do not seek it out until a problem arises. I've included it at the beginning of this program because it's a wonderful way to embody your body. Most exercise programs are about getting the most out of your workouts in terms of intensity, strength, and cardiovascular fitness. How about getting the most out of life? Ultramarathons are useless to those who cannot get up and down from a chair without discomfort. Humans are reactive animals, waiting until the last possible moment to implement necessary changes. Feldenkrais offers proactive, prescriptive means for avoiding chronic problems. Plus it feels great to practice.

That's because Feldenkrais tapped into something primal in human nature. Movement began the moment you were conceived. An assembly of neurons has created cortical maps with innumerable connections helping to create your identity, the structures of who you are. Embedded in your identity are the emotional-cognitive aspects of personality. This includes the way you move through the world: your gait, posture, speed, strength, and subtle but inevitable imbalances. These are as much a part of *you* as any thought firing inside of your head. You can change your mind; you can change your body. Most importantly you can change both, simultaneously. In order to accomplish this, you have to work with your nervous system. Better put: you are your nervous system (and so much more, though it truly begins here).

Outside of physics and movement, Feldenkrais was a keen cultural observer. He knew breathing to be an essential component of health. But in general we pay little attention to our autonomic faculties. Too much stimulation keeps us in a state of constant distraction. While Feldenkrias took no issue with certain forms of speed—basic instinctual movements are often by necessity rapid, such as jumping out of the way of a vehicle or reacting to an attacker—Feldenkrais believed humanity's perpetual state of hurry to be tragic. Somatic education is slow. If you're going to retrain movement, your mind must be at ease. Moving from sympathetic to parasympathetic mode allows the information to take hold, resulting in constructive change. Important details are lost when you're not paying attention.

Reversibility is an important component of physical and mental training: use it or lose it, as the saying goes. We know that our bodies lose muscle composition after just a few weeks of not training. Similar results occur in our brains—one study showed a noticeable amount of decreased blood flow after just ten days off cardiovascular activity.[11] For Feldenkrais, calming your nervous system is not a once in a while practice. To make lasting changes you must regularly quiet your mind and still your body. Such changes are measurable. For example, increased gray matter has been found in the brains of consistent meditators, leading to decreased levels of stress and increased memory.[12] You won't need an fMRI scan to recognize the benefits, however. Spending time in these reflective states while practicing subtle movements will aid you in a later chapter when we stand up to strengthen our muscles and build our resolve. For now, lie down.

THE PROGRAM: FELDENKRAIS

Exercise #1: Refined Articulations

Begin lying on your back. Ideally, you'll be on the floor, on a carpet, or yoga mat. This is also possible to practice in bed, though this creates problems since we associate our bed with sleeping. If you experience discomfort, place a yoga bolster or rolled blanket under your knees to alleviate pressure from your lower back; likewise, use a thin pillow for your neck. I find the best success when my body can lie flat on the ground. The surface increases my awareness of bodily tension, which informs me of what I need to release.

Close your eyes. Ambient music might be nice, though for this section I prefer silence. Take ten deep breaths, allowing your exhale to be longer than your inhale. Feel your body soften into the floor; let the ground support you completely. By paying attention to your breathing you should be able to slow down the rapidity of thoughts as well.

After ten breaths, bring your attention to your right foot. Is it turned out or pointing straight up? Don't alter the position; simply notice where it is when relaxed. Then activate your big toe by stretching it slightly away from the others. Go down the line: second toe, third toe, etc. Can you move your toes individually? Instead of trying to move the entire foot at once, focus on the subtle sensations of each toe. Can you differentiate the second from the third toe enough to feel it activate? Even without moving your toes at all, can you *feel* each one as a separate digit?

Spend a minute on each toe. Observe if you're clenching any part of your body. It's very common to transfer tension. Notice if your eyes feel stressed behind your closed eyelids. Remember, any movement, including the movement of thinking, activates your nervous system. Do your best to keep your attention on your toes, with the rest of your body in a state of complete relaxation.

After you've gone down the line, slowly spread and clench all five toes at once. Observe how little movement in your ankle joint and calves this requires; at first, it might seem like a lot. Once you've done this a few times you're going to move up to your right ankle. Begin by noticing the sensation of it: its heaviness on the floor, the weight of the joint. Then slowly rotate your ankle to the left and right, ten times in each direction. Don't aim for a stretch, however. Just let its natural range of motion unfold without exhibiting too much effort. After you've done this ten times, take a few deep breaths, allowing your body to return to a state of total relaxation.

Head to your right knee and right hip joints next. Follow the same procedures. Don't aim for a stretch, especially with your knee. These are extremely small articulations. Do your best to not think about how much you are or are not doing. In terms of your nervous system, you're accomplishing plenty. You're training your brain to observe extremely small movement patterns, which is going to make a huge difference in how you relate to every other movement or exercise you do next.

After you finish your right leg, repeat the entire sequence on your left leg.

Exercise #2: Twist and (Don't) Shout

Lying on your back, bend your knees and place your feet on the floor, with your arms extended next to your hips. Press into your forearms and slowly lift your hips into a bridge on your inhale. Feel the entirety of your spine lift from the floor, beginning with your lower back, then mid-back, and then up to your shoulders. On your exhale, retrace that pattern until your sacrum returns to the ground. Repeat this ten times, increasing the lift of your hips with each repetition.

After completing a set of ten repetitions, extend your arms straight out to the sides with your palms down. Keep both shoulders on the ground as you drop your knees to the right and left in a "windshield wiper" movement. This twisting motion should be gentle; don't thrust your body around. Use your forearms pressing into the floor to stabilize your shoulders and neck muscles. Let the knees drop to one side on your exhale, using your inhale to return them back to center.

After eight rounds, roll your entire body side to side. Let your knees drop over to the right, then feel your left shoulder lift, taking your arm all the way over to the right side so that you end up in a "fetal" position. Then roll to the other side. Try to be soft and supple, not allowing momentum to propel you. Envision your body as a slow pendulum easefully floating left to right.

Complete eight repetitions until you begin rolling all the way over onto your hands and knees. Once you come up into a table position, lower back and roll to the other side. Completing four rounds to each side, pause on your hands and knees, tuck your toes, and lift your hips into the air into a Downward Dog posture. Take five deep breaths lengthening your spine, then walk your hands back to your feet and take five more breaths hanging over your legs in a forward bend, with your knees soft and neck and jaw relaxed.

This exercise is designed to move you from a lying to a standing position. After five breaths, soften your knees generously and roll up to standing, imagining each vertebra lengthening on your way up. Notice how your body feels with your eyes closed for five more breaths, then blink your eyes open and prepare for Exercise #3.

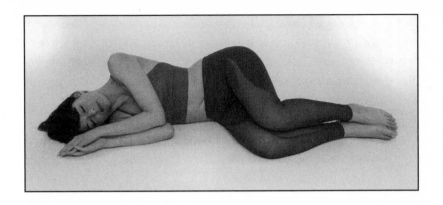

Exercise #3: Going Flamingo

In the first exercise, you investigated your toes. In the next chapter, you're going to explore your feet. Thanks to the evolutionary adaption of bipedalism, so much depends on them. They are our connection to the ground, but rarely do we discuss exercising our feet. That's tragic , as most of us have some imbalances, which often begin here. In many ways proprioception, the internal guidance of how we navigate our environment, also starts here.

With your eyes closed, place your feet hip-width apart. Keep your knees soft, palms facing forward, and shoulders drawn down your back, with your head elongating toward the ceiling. Notice any subtle shift in your ankle joints; even in stillness there is subtle movement. After five breaths holding this stance, gently shift the weight forward and back ten times. Then shift your weight side to side the same number of repetitions. Observing every nuanced movement in your feet and ankles, circulate your body in a clockwise direction five times; then move counter-clockwise. After you've finished these centration exercises, pause in what feels to be the middle of both feet, with your body's weight spread out on all four corners of both feet, for another five breaths. Slowly open your eyes.

Soften your right knee and lift your left foot three inches off the ground. If possible, straighten your left leg by flexing your left foot. Your knees are parallel; you're not trying to lift your foot very high.

This is more about feeling the distribution of weight and balance in your right foot. Hold for five breaths, then repeat on your left side. If this is especially challenging, hold onto a chair or table beside you until your ankle has the strength to hold the position.

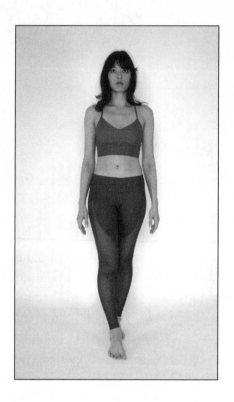

Once you've accomplished this, walk ten paces forward as if you are on a tightrope, placing your right foot directly in front of your left, then continuing in that fashion. Observe every small movement—the rolling of your foot right to left, or vice-versa; any gripping in your toes; any pain in your heel or forefoot. Try to be as soft and relaxed in your torso as possible. When you complete ten steps, turn around and walk back, or, for a more challenging option, walk backwards. Once you feel proficient in this movement, try it with your eyes closed to challenge your balance.

Remember, none of these exercises are "hard" in modern fitness terminology. The real challenge is refining your awareness and calming your nervous system to prepare you for bigger, more challenging movements—or, to simply focus. We spend most of our days moving while paying little attention to our breathing, gait, sitting posture, and the myriad ways we carry ourselves. These exercises are designed to make you hyper-aware of the subtle aspects of movement. This is just as, if not more, important than the following chapters. While I'm a fan of numerous movements, tuning in to what my body is feeling (and why) is critical information needed for optimal health. Treat these exercises with as much detail as anything ahead.

Now that you're tuned in, let's get your heart rate up. Sensory awareness is slow, but not everything in life is meant to be chill. To start things off, let's begin again with your feet.

Chapter 5

Pump Up the Volume

"I just run. I run in a void. Or maybe I should put it the other way:
I run in order to *acquire* a void."

—Haruki Murakami, *What I Talk About
When I Talk About Running*

WHAT ARE WE DOING IT FOR?

Temescal Canyon Road is a moderate incline from the Pacific Ocean
to the beginning of the sixty-seven-mile Backbone Trail through
the Santa Monica Mountains. While the trail actually begins in the
adjacent Will Rogers State Historic Park, Temescal is where the terrain gets serious. Since moving to Los Angeles, it has been my go-to
hike and run.

I arrive at seven on a cool July morning. The infamous "June
gloom" has, for the past two summers, overstayed its welcome.
I'm thankful for the cloud cover given last week's Corral Canyon
hike in ninety-degree heat. For over two decades, hiking has been
an essential in my life, mostly because to me, there's no "exercise"
involved. The fact that I'm working out is secondary to the joy of
climbing mountains. Throughout my twenties I'd scramble, picking various streams and rivers in Northwestern New Jersey to sprint
up, skipping from rock to rock, using my toes to grip wet surfaces

and test my balance. In my thirties, I migrated forty minutes north of Manhattan on weekends, alternating between walks and sprints at Anthony Wayne State Park. My forties have been devoted to trail running, focusing on longer, sustained paces rather than quick bursts of frenetic energy followed by oxygen gasps.

It's not that I'm leaving quick bursts behind—we'll get to those shortly, as they offer wonderful conditioning and will be your workout for this modality. On this July morning I show up to challenge myself on one of the topics of this book: to disrupt my normal fitness routine, as well as prove to myself that I'm capable of doing things I thought I'd never accomplish.

Mindset influences performance. If your first response to a challenge is "no," then how do you expect to grow? Your nervous system is the catalyst for movement, yet it also receives sensory information from your environment to understand how to move through it. Deciding on novel means of doing so changes your relationship to your surroundings, just as it changes how you comprehend your body.

I've long had a love/mostly hate relationship with running. About ten years prior, I tore my right labrum training for a half-marathon in Brooklyn's Prospect Park. A few months of physical therapy had me moving normally, though I wouldn't run again for two years. As most of my conditioning involved yoga and strength training, I noticed myself becoming winded climbing subway stairs. My heart and brain suffered from a lack of cardiovascular activity. I hopped on a treadmill, felt pretty good, and immediately began envisioning the half-marathon again. A few months back in Prospect Park and—hello torn left meniscus. This time I put myself through therapy. For two and a half years I partook in other forms of cardio—studio and outdoor cycling and basketball. One day a clumsy defensive player clipped my left thigh. Less than a year after having had cancer surgery at UCLA, I returned to have a surgeon slice out a sizable portion of my left meniscus.

You can imagine how all these factors would keep me from ever running again. My surgeon informed me that my running (and jumping) days were over. I acquiesced. When I avoid running it's easy to make excuses. *I can't, my doctor says so.* Something irked me, however. How could I abandon what our bodies are built for just as I was entering middle age? Could I really envision another forty, hopefully fifty years on this planet without trotting from time to time? Centenarians finish marathons. At forty was I really calling it quits?

I investigated the conditions leading to my injuries. I broke my right femur when I was eleven, laid up in bed for three months in traction and a full body cast, as if out of a seventeenth-century torture manual. (Doctors have since recognized that moving an injured limb aids recovery.) This break often leads to labrum problems, as well as compensation in weight distribution between legs. I'm shocked that my left knee lasted as long as it did given that I also broke my right ankle twice. Factor in that both of my running injuries occurred in winter while training in forty-degree temperatures. These puzzle pieces left me wondering if running is the real problem.

In *Born to Run*, Christopher McDougall discusses an oft-missing element in modern running: fun. Previously I was so focused on attaining a goal that I forgot that part of the story. As an ultra-competitive species we've monetized an evolutionary adaptation. Race times equal sponsors. Or we've quantified it by thinking a run has to be eight thousand steps. There's nothing wrong with earning a living from your passion or having goals. When those eclipse sheer pleasure, we have to ask ourselves why we do what we do. I realized that what I really loathe is running on treadmills and flat surfaces. So I decided to run up hills.

Given Temescal's proximity to urban Los Angeles, I'm surprised by how few people I pass along the way. On this particular morning, that equals one woman on the way up and a couple with a dog during my descent. I begin the climb with a light jog. Temescal has a quick ascent followed by, depending if you're heading north or east to Will Rogers, a series of climbs and drops that will be your return route. I decide on the series and turn left. Pushing my threshold during the initial phase, I regulate my breathing going up and down. As expected, I'm winded on the first push, though given my slower pace I last a lot longer than expected. A brief walk and I jump back in. ("Running is really just jumping, springing from one foot to another," McDougall writes.[1]) By the time I reach the first peak my lungs are wide open. Whatever sense of being winded I had dissipates. I head through a thicket of brush, scraping my shins. I reach the bottom to start another climb when a quadruped scurries off the path into the sharp tangles of plants twenty feet ahead. I pause, damning myself for not having purchased pepper spray. Just the previous day I'd read about five new mountain lion cubs born in these very hills. I slowly turn the corner, recalling that most animals want nothing to do with a lumbering, gasping six-three representative of *Homo sapiens*. I easily reach my normal turnaround; I eye the next peak. Runner's high is going strong; I sprint up another two levels before turning back. The following week I reach the final peak more quickly, straddling the sky with only the sounds of bird and cloud whisking along my back.

Like many others, I'd subscribed to the notion that the human body is not designed to run. Hasn't evolution screwed us by injecting so many foot problems? With pervasive ankle and knee injuries, lower back and shoulder tightness, why would we believe accelerating our bipedal tendencies is beneficial? Up to 70 percent of runners are injured every year.[2] How good can it really be for us?

Very, if we're smart about it. The myth of faulty design is yet another failure of common wisdom rooted in marketing hype. In the last chapter we learned what it takes to get up off the ground. Now that we're standing, let's consider the most underappreciated part of our body: our feet. To get our heart rate elevated and skin lubricated, we start at the foundation.

BOTTOMS UP

Why a group of hairy mammals stopped dragging their knuckles to walk on two feet might never be known. We know this adaptation occurred slowly, and is not exclusive to us. Bears, kangaroos, and chimps are bipedal, at least part of the time. We did master the style, although we're losing mastery as we slouch all day. Think about survival strategies from being bipedal: we can see further into the distance, which informs us of approaching danger, such as predators or storms. We can also spot our tribe more easily, increasing communication potential. Over that time our feet have slowly restructured. A quarter of our body's muscles are in our feet; each foot boasts thirty-three joints. Yet we rarely consider the complexity and dexterity of these limbs, given that they spend most hours stuffed into shoes. Imagine how much sensory input would be lost if you wore mittens each day, every day. That's essentially what we're doing to our feet.

Ten thousand years ago, sandals lifted us a few millimeters off the ground. While a wonderful technology that saves our skin from sharp objects, they're tragic for sensory input. Fast-forward another four-and-a-half millennia and moccasins hit the runway, creating a further barrier between sole and environment. Incredibly, this remained the general form of footwear for eons. Sure, heels emerged centuries ago, as did all sorts of boots and contraptions. Check out a race or basketball game from the middle of the last century and you'll witness men lumbering around in canvas Converse sneakers not that much different from moccasins. Shoes were minimalist for quite some time.

What was most likely a response to plantar fasciitis—plantar fascia is a thick, triangular band of tissue connecting your toes with your heel; fasciitis is a catchall for any problem with that band—someone padded the heel of running shoes as a quick fix. Instead of striking pavement, we'll strike an air pocket! Problem is we generally don't strike with our heels unless forced to do so by elevating it above the rest of our foot. Over forty-five million years (roughly four million when considering our lineage), quadrupeds evolved to bipedalism. Within the span of a decade, Nike tricked us into believing nature got it all wrong. By 2018, the athletic footwear industry in America is predicted to top $84 billion.[3] It makes sense that shoe companies want to protect their investment by making us believe we need them.

Try this experiment if you want to understand what's going on when you run in a heeled shoe. Take off your shoes and socks, ideally on a carpeted floor to absorb some of the impact. Bend your knees and jump up a few inches (recall that running is a series of jumps). Notice how your feet naturally land. Then soften your knees again and jump an inch or two and land on your heels. Don't jump any higher; you'll feel it right away. Now consider that this is what you're doing, again and again and again, when you heel strike. Five hundred miles and another hundred and fifty bucks later another podiatrist awaits.

We imagine technology as unerringly progressive, but we do well to remember there's always a sacrifice. If the technology addresses a symptom and not the cause, how will you unearth the root? Statins and antacids serve this role in our diet: eat whatever you'd like and take this pill. Padded shoes and orthotics are statins for our feet, and therefore for our entire bodies. Even chronic headaches can be caused by immobile ankles. Full-body nerve health suffers when we scrunch our toes into shoes. Seniors often fall due to a lost neuronal connection between their brain and feet. Combine this with avoiding impact through running or strength training and osteoporosis risk greatly increases—55 percent of Americans over age fifty have low bone mass, equating to 1.5 million fractures every year.[4] Our bodies need to be jostled a bit to stay firm. This begins with our feet.

Heeled shoes restrict your range of motion in a number of joints, not just your ankles. To adjust to the seemingly innocuous millimeters that heeled shoes raise your body from the ground, you walk as if going downhill.[5] Tight ankles create a variety of mismatches, including valgus knee collapse (the knees are twisted in toward your midline), collapsed arches, plantar fasciitis, and bone spurs. These conditions are often treated through ice, rest, and orthotics, none of which address structural damage. Forget running, this happens just by walking. Factor in impact peak—a spike in force when your heels slam into the ground—and you've just sent a shockwave from calcaneus to head. The benefits of heel striking, including a lengthened stride and less stress on your calf muscles and Achilles tendon, pale in comparison to damage being done. Heel strikers are more likely to experience repetitive stress injuries than barefoot runners.[6]

Many students and clients with foot problems cite years of misuse. An hour of preventive care in a yoga class is better than nothing. Yet if the rest of the day is spent in shoes, the problems will only be perpetuated. Cultures create norms; sneakers and shoes are fetish and fashion objects. I simply can't imagine sacrificing my health for such reasons. The minimalist shoe industry is relatively small but growing—some runners consider the "barefoot phase" over, which is a shame. That means marketing once again wins. If you care about your body, investigate how you treat your feet. Your training will not be optimal without addressing them first. This does not imply that you must *always* go barefoot; I don't rock Vibrams or Inov8s when going out to dinner. Spend as much time as possible barefoot, and wear minimal shoes whenever you can.

Now that my public service announcement is over, let's talk about what to do with your feet. As this program focuses on training you can do anywhere, we're soon going to discuss high-intensity interval training, which accounts for half of my personal cardio. I don't want to gloss over running, considering that 541,000 people finished marathons in 2013. The health benefits of running are well documented. As we're all born to run we need to understand why running is such an important component of being human. Besides obvious cardiovascular benefits, running boosts another critical component of brain and body fitness. To learn more, we return to school.

TIME TO WAKE UP

In his book *Spark*, John J. Ratey visits Naperville Central High School in a Chicago suburb. Budget cuts around the country have resulted in schools eliminating arts and physical education programs to focus on competitive subjects like science and mathematics. Naperville officials felt this to be misguided, however, as optimal functioning requires that we feed our brain with movement. As a result, Zero Hour was born.

An optional before-school program, Zero Hour students gather at 7:10 a.m. for a brief warm-up before heading to the track. Four loops are timed; the physical education teacher straps each student with a heart monitor, hoping that everyone maintains a heart rate of

185 during their mile-long run. Olympian times are irrelevant. For example, one girl clocked in at just over ten minutes, maintaining a heart rate of 191. No records broken, yet she's giving herself a serious leg up before first period. Naperville physical education teacher Neil Duncan aims for 80-90 percent of VO_2 max, ensuring quality neurological functioning.

VO_2 max refers to maximal oxygen uptake, the true gem of aerobic exercise and the main reason so many people strap a fitness tracker around their wrists, beyond counting steps. Steps are important, but how you walk (or run) those steps is more telling. VO_2 max is relative to your weight; the more oxygen you can inhale and transport around to your muscles, the better your endurance. You want to increase endurance while inhaling as much oxygen as possible to help create functional changes in your body, allowing for increased blood flow, as well as to amplify the power and capacity of your aerobic system. Aerobic activity also optimizes out-of-balance bodily systems. All of these reasons are great for your heart as well as your brain. For Naperville students, this translated as a 17 percent increase in reading and comprehension; classmates choosing to doze showed only a 10.2 percent increase. A seven percent difference between these groups might not sound like a lot until you consider how competitive college entrance exams are. That extra hour of huffing it pays off major dividends.

Guidance counselors at the school caught on and started stacking the hardest classes of the day during first and second period. Students not only self-reported major declines in crankiness levels, but also their test scores soared, especially in challenging subjects. This goes a long way toward overturning the myth of the all-night cramming session fueled by coffee and carbohydrate-heavy junk foods. Sleep well and run and you greatly increase your chances at acing a test. Stay up all night tossing back lattes and fries and there's little chance you'll retain much of anything. Sure, you might memorize just enough to pass. Give it a week and see where the data went.

Those of us in the workforce might not need to study for tests anymore, though who can't use a bump in performance? Aerobic activity—not only running, but swimming, bicycling, and cross-country skiing—is helpful for memory. Once your heart rate soars, sympathetic stimulation of your fight-flight-freeze system kicks in, which is one reason running helps me with anxiety attacks. You literally outrun fear. Your adrenal glands pump epinephrine and norepinephrine, which along with dopamine are collectively known as catecholamines, to help meet the metabolic demands being placed on your body. Blood floods active muscle cells. Your metabolic system gets a boost. Anxiety disappears, or, as Kelly McGonigal puts it, you reframe the focus of stress for a beneficial purpose.

We all know about the obesity epidemic in America and, increasingly, many other countries that adopt carbohydrate- and sugar-heavy diets. Combined with better eating habits, aerobic exercise is key for losing visceral fat, increasing lean weight, and lowering your risk of heart disease and type 2 diabetes. Lower risk is the catchall: early death, stroke, falling, depression, metabolic syndrome, and a variety of cancers are all implicated. Better cognitive functioning is especially apparent in elder populations as well as in teenagers, though this appears true for people of any age.

While the benefits of cardiovascular training are endless and essential, perhaps no other movement form is susceptible to overtraining. Chasing the runner's high can be a daily occupation. Marathon fanatics push their bodies to the edge. This is fine—endurance running offers wonderful benefits if your body can handle it—but you've got to regenerate just as intensely, giving your body and brain a break from the excessive stimulation of oxygen uptake. The forthcoming exercises are complementary to the other four workouts in this section, especially if you're not getting your heart rate up already. For those that already are, I'd focus on the more relaxing prescriptions ahead.

Yet it's hard to give up the runner's high. This indescribable state is also known as flow. There are many ways to achieve flow states; my personal favorite is reading, though I do love a good running bliss. One important requirement for flow, as understood by psychologist Mihaly Csíkszentmihályi, is to love what you're doing. Runners certainly love running. Checking in with *why* you love running is important, as this is part of recognizing when you're overtraining.

Obsessively maintaining a certain body weight or self-image is the physical equivalent of orthorexia, an eating disorder defined by an unhealthy need for particular foods. The eater becomes paralyzed by indecision over what is healthy and what is not; at extreme ends they'll limit their diet to one or two items. Likewise, I know people that *only* run. Remember, variety is key. If endurance training is your mojo, run ahead. Introducing other aspects of fitness—intense Tabatas, resistance training, or (and I'd argue, especially) yoga and meditation—is crucial in balancing your movement lifestyle.

Throughout literature, running is probably the most celebrated exercise. We can thank the high for that. In his memoir, Japanese novelist Haruki Murakami discusses his emotional connection to endurance running. An overweight, jazz club-owning smoker in the seventies, he eventually found clarity and meaning in life running ultra-marathons. As for why he runs, he writes, "When I'm criticized unjustly (from my viewpoint, at least), or when someone I'm sure will understand me doesn't, I go running for a little longer than usual. By running long it's like I can physically exhaust that portion of my discontent."[7]

Running also helps Murakami in other ways, including the fact that it helps him identify his limits and try to break past them, ultimately growing stronger, and it also helps turn his angers and frustrations inwards as a means of improving himself. That clarity, the refusal to give up, is an honorable trait. In many ways it ensured our survival: persistence hunting required that our ancestors move dozens of miles a day to exhaust and capture their prey. Marathons were mandatory, not lifestyle choices. There is something primal in our quest to cover vast expanses of terrain, to get lost in the rhythm of our breath, the cadence of our foot strikes on the gravel and trail. By being smart and dedicated to our discipline, there's no reason we can't run well into our nineties. We only have to treat the machinery of our bodies and brains properly.

Then again, some people would rather not imagine putting in a hundred or even twenty miles a week. Different formats require different temperaments. This book might involve disruption, yet it also honors personal tastes. For some, getting the heart rate up is its own reward. For those who love quicker bouts of intensity, Tabatas are a wonderful invention.

FULL VOLUME

It's no easy chore to have a protocol named after you. Izumi Tabata credits Kouichi Irisawa, head coach of the Japanese National Speed Skating Team, for inventing the technique bearing his name. Tabata, a dean at Ritsumeikan University, published the paper in 1996 that made quick, high-intensity bouts of cardio famous. Unlike many fads that are forgotten tomorrow, this one has only grown in the two decades since its publication. In fact, in 2013 Tabata co-trademarked an official workout with Universal Pictures. His twenty-minute format has not caught on, but the four-minute bouts of intense exercise he initially prescribed certainly did.

High-intensity interval training (HIIT) is a general term for any activity that involves giving it your all for a brief duration, then either resting or actively recovering before doing it again. This format is a wonderful companion to running. There is evidence that HIIT improves endurance training[8], which makes sense, given how rapidly you're feeding your body oxygen. This physiological hack is felt any time you're startled. Imagine if that quadruped I stumbled across on the trail, which I'm guessing was a coyote, was actually the mama mountain lion of those new cubs. And she's not scurrying; she's staring right at me. Better believe I'm about to fly, one evolutionary purpose of the fight-flight-freeze mechanism. Translating this to exercise, by priming the pump on that system, over and over in quick bursts, you're exploiting one of the most beneficial forms of exercise, even if our ancestors would never have dreamed of it beyond life-or-death situations. Then again, who knows when the first sprints began? We certainly don't have a monopoly on fun.

High-intensity workouts are also mentally engaging. With Tabatas you've got twenty seconds to focus on form, power, and speed. By the time you've caught your breath, you're full throttle in the next round. Aerobic exercise has shown improvements in executive function, attentional control, processing speed, and visuospatial skills, in addition to focus.[9] While I love trail running, a four-minute charge during the day as a break from my desk is a wonderful way to refocus.

Yet Tabatas are not without controversy. Trainers refute the protocol's metabolic claims. These mostly involve arguments over the quickest way to lose weight. As stated earlier, that is not the focus of this book. I'm more concerned with cognitive functioning. Without doubt, this format aids in that quest.

THE PROGRAM: CARDIOVASCULAR TRAINING

Tabatas are intense bursts of movement. For each exercise you'll perform the movement for twenty seconds and take a ten-second break. Do not sit down; you'll need the time to recover and catch your breath. Perform each movement eight times, with eight breaks. After you finish one set, rest for two minutes and move on to the next exercise. This entire section should be performed in eighteen minutes. To time it you can download a free tabata stopwatch on your phone or tablet. If possible, avoid using your watch, as looking down at your wrist is a distraction. Setting your device on the ground or a table allows you to view time without breaking stride.

Exercise #1: Driving Lunges

During this movement you'll alternate which leg is in front, so by the end you'll have performed four lunges on each side. Alternate each round.

1. Begin with your right foot forward and your left leg back in a lunging position. Your left hand is inside of your right foot; your right hand is either outside of your right foot or reaching down the side of your body. I suggest being on your fingertips for quicker release. Draw your shoulders down your back, lengthen your sternum forward, and gaze straight ahead.

2. You'll drive your left knee up toward your chest as you stand up on your right leg. It's a kinetic burst. Don't go too fast to begin; focus on form. Is your left knee driving toward the left side of your chest? Are your shoulders drawn down as you stand up? Do you feel your body weight evenly spread out on all four corners of your right foot? Is your right knee slightly bent? You'll want to hit all of these markers. After you drive the knee up, step back into the lunge with your hands returning to the ground. Repeat for twenty seconds.

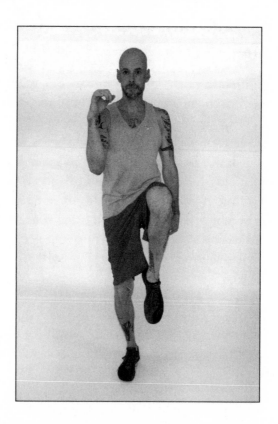

3. To perform a plyometric version, which raises the intensity level, as you drive your left knee up jump off the ground with your right foot. When you land, your left leg immediately returns to a lunge.

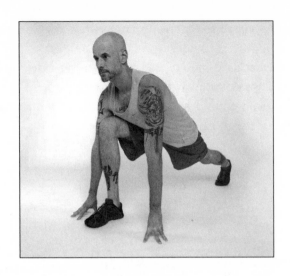

4. Stand up and switch sides. If you perform a plyometric version on one side, make sure to do the same on the other. You can also perform one round plyometric, the next without jumping.

Exercise #2: Squat Taps

I'm a daily squatter. I do a minimum of twenty bodyweight squats every single day as part of a warm-up routine. Sometimes I perform them right out of bed to wake up my legs. Most days I do many more squats, sometimes in the hundreds. This squat involves tapping the ground with your hand to create an element of length in your torso.

Important note: Make sure that your knees line up over the middle of your feet. Valgus knee has detrimental effects over time. Likewise, varus knee—when the knees extend too far away from the midline—leads to chronic problems. You might consider warming up with a few simple squats to focus on form before beginning the tabatas.

1. Stand with your feet shoulder's width apart.
2. Step to the right with your right foot and drop into a squat. As you're dropping down, tap your left hand between your feet, creating a slight twist in your upper body. You want to look

straight ahead so that you're not either twisting your left knee or dropping your chest too far to the right.

3. Stand back up and repeat on the other side. Each time you stand, make sure to drive your body's energy upwards from your heels. Avoid being on the balls of your toes when you move through this sequence.

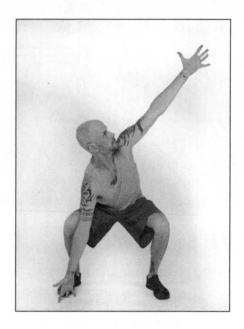

Exercise #3: Roundhouse Squats

Now that your hips are warmed up let's keep squatting. While squatting seems like just one movement, there are numerous ways to move in and out of them. This is one of my favorites, as it creates a large range of motion in your hip joints. In martial arts, a roundhouse kick is a semicircular movement that involves explosive power. You won't be throwing any kicks, but as you progress with this movement you'll gain more power driving from your heels up to the standing position.

1. Begin standing with your feet shoulder's width apart.
2. Step to the right with your right foot and drop into a squat.

As you stand, lift your right knee toward your left shoulder, then circle your leg toward your right shoulder. Don't focus on how high your leg goes as much as the rotation as you swing your leg across your midline, with the hip ending in external rotation. Return to the squat.

3. Repeat on the left side. Alternate sides each time.

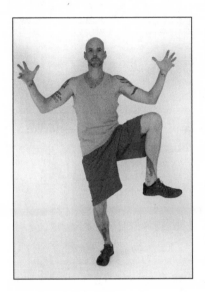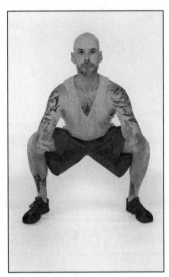

Chapter 6

Resistance is Not Futile

"Learning coordination is a matter of training the nervous system and not a question of training muscles."

—Bruce Lee, *Tao of Jeet Kune Do*

BEYOND FORMS

Of all forms portrayed in society, "muscular" is the most lauded. Lean muscle, ripped muscle, bulky muscle—anything cut or large or cut *and* large will do. Yet we're oddly particular about what kinds of muscles inspire us. Toned abs is a big one. Legs and rear for the women; chest and biceps for the men; and defined shoulders, regardless of gender, all catch our attention. How about a toned flexor hallucis longus? Get real. A ripped quadratus lumborum? Well, many do get ripped, or at least tight, which leads to rips in the form of hernias. Humans obsess over certain muscles at the expense of others, forgetting that our entire body is a support system of itself. For example, triceps own more real estate than biceps, but guys love to show the latter. The result is an imbalance: weak and tight muscles vying for the attention given to over-trained areas.

A fascination with size is cultural. In the nineteenth century strongmen appeared on vaudeville stages to display how much weight they could toss around. Around the time my great-grandfather was leaving Russia, his fellow countrymen were filling circular molds with iron to create what would become known as kettlebells. As early as 1878, men were competing to swing, press, snatch, and jerk the heaviest weights. Eighteen years later, weightlifting achieved Olympic status in Athens.[1] While lifting protocol has evolved, the events only go in one direction: bigger. In the 1960s, powerlifting became a separate sport from the Olympics. This opened the door for Jack LaLanne and Arnold Schwarzenegger to dominate a burgeoning fitness industry. While other cultures have always practiced various ways of working out, Americans perfected "fitness" as separate from a movement-based lifestyle, for better *and* worse. With numerous citizens now sitting at desks for a third of their life, their bodies and brains have suffered the costs of stagnancy. Exercise became a necessary balance to sedentary working conditions, a struggle many face daily.

My health-conscious father was a devoted member of Jack LaLanne's gym. I grew up with a makeshift gym in my basement, thanks to my dad's incessant exercise. A handful of free weights; a creaky eighties-era multi-purpose machine for chest, back, and leg exercises; a sit-up bench; and a punching bag were all present (my dad's favorite sport is boxing). Being a sports fanatic, I didn't grow up lifting weights. Running around a diamond and chasing fly balls was more appealing. But I certainly went through cycles of lifting, especially through high school and college. Besides working in computer operations for over four decades, my father ran his company's gym. Going there was an early bonding ritual for us.

My enthusiasm for resistance training has waxed and waned. During college, it dominated my free time alongside basketball and volleyball. Five days a week I'd spend an hour doing circuits: back and biceps one day, chest and triceps the next, and legs following. My relationship to resistance is much different today. While I still go heavy twice a week, I prefer to load with a VIPR and kettlebells. Free weights are best, though if I use a machine, wobbly cables are more realistic to real-life movements than machines that force perfect execution. Sure, you'll spot train one action really well, but how often do we organically repeat *any* movement the same way? I'd rather be thrown off balance so that I have to constantly recalibrate. Such resistance is truer to life.

My favorite piece of equipment is my body, however. Like language, movement is infinite. With writing you're given a set number of letters that result in a staggering possibility of results. The same is true of your body. Your only restriction is a lack of creativity. Unfortunately, I've watched many people fall into the same resistance rut. Monday is back day when I do this many reps of this; Tuesday is chest and I cycle through this; and so on. As stated, any movement is better than none. Yet creating a large movement vocabulary and continually mixing and matching—constantly creating new narratives and stories, thereby creating new neural pathways—is the best scenario. Make sure to explore a number of rotations throughout your entire range of motion. Exercise your core while also working out your back and quadriceps, or chest and triceps. Spot training has a purpose—specific competitive goals are a different story—but it can take all the fun out of movement. We just weren't built to do thirty repetitions of any movement every Wednesday morning.

BEGIN WITH FORM

Just as many people don't learn to run—they just go out and do it—the same occurs with resistance training. That too is dangerous. Form is key. Sure, on occasion I'll see a guy pull down the bar *behind* his head. Old habits die hard. More commonly, I'll watch students move into planks and side plank postures with their shoulders a few inches behind their hands, setting them up for all sorts of shoulder issues. The body is like any structure: it needs to be solid but not stiff, firm with room to yield. If you stop with your shoulders two inches behind your wrists, that can often lead to rotator cuff impingement.

Proper form is essential for the development of neuromuscular facilitation. Contracting your muscles, whether a concentric (the muscle shortens), eccentric (lengthens), or isometric (static tension with no change in length) movement, is a function controlled by your brain. Focused repetition from brain to muscle creates good form. Like riding a bicycle, burpees (also known as squat thrusts) require a lot of thought and patience at first, but over time they become second nature. Learning good form at the beginning is essential. Muscle memory is like any other learned behavior. If your form is poor you have to undo inefficiencies while simultaneously integrating proper mechanics. This is harder to accomplish than getting it right from the outset. For example, I've watched trainers teach clients handstands like a cheerleader: start standing, throw your hands down, kick up near a wall, hope balance happens. If you use momentum instead of muscular contraction to perform a handstand, you've failed before you've even begun.

Balancing your resistance program is also important. As mentioned, we tend to focus on certain areas and neglect others. Due to environmental conditions, such as sitting too much and poor posture, we undertrain and don't stretch enough. Our body consists of opposing forces, with one muscle or group relying on another—take hamstrings, for instance. Hamstrings tend to be tight, as you know if you have difficulty tying your shoes. If you need to sit down to tie them there's a mechanical issue. Stretching is key. Other muscles that tend to be tight include pectorals, upper trapezius (hello texting), and calf muscles.

Then there's weak muscle. Abdominal muscles often fall into this category; combine underperforming abs with a tight QL (quadratus lumborum) and you have a mechanical recipe for disaster. External shoulder rotators, rear deltoids, and mid- and lower-trapezius muscles fall into this category as well. Outside of abs, these muscles are rarely the focus of magazine covers. Most people don't know where their QL is located, but when I touch them there they immediately recognize a problem. Becoming an anatomical genius is not required. Yet ignoring weaknesses and tightness while overtraining certain groups will catch up to you, quickly. If something feels off, it probably is. Your brain is sending you a warning. Listen to it.

Enter mental health. Resistance is essential for a well-rounded body and brain. With all the exciting research in aerobic exercise, yoga, and meditation, resistance training receives less attention, even though it's the go-to for many fitness enthusiasts. Since resistance does not get your heart rate into the maximal zone, or slow you down into parasympathetic mode, researchers have not looked as thoroughly into its neurological effects. But that's changing. There is evidence that resistance training helps in neurogenesis.[2] Ladder-climbing rats with weights tied to their tails showed sizable increases in BDNF. Three years after this study suggested weight training can also help humans, researchers tested healthy college-aged men to verify that yes, throwing around iron has a similar effect on our brain as it does that of our rodent cousins.[3] (Mice and humans share roughly 96–97 percent DNA.)

Remember, BDNF aids memory. A study of women aged sixty-five to seventy-five who lifted weights twice a week for one year showed marked improvements in reducing lesions or holes in their brains' white matter over groups that lifted once a week or only stretched and practiced balancing exercises.[4] As we age, such lesions take over our brain's white matter, reducing the connectivity between different neural regions. While some lesions are benign, others lead to strokes and other diseases. They also affect memory. This study suggests that not only is lifting weights helpful in retaining our ability to remember as we age, but frequency matters also.

Don't think you need to go all-out, all the time, however. Another study found promising results in episodic memory from just a single resistance training session.[5] A team at Georgia Tech had participants view ninety photos on a computer screen. One group performed fifty leg extensions while the other had the machine move their legs. The group that performed the extensions themselves exhibited a 10 percent increase in accuracy two days later when returning to recall the photos. Interestingly, the resistance-training group also exhibited increased levels of norepinephrine in their saliva, which plays a role in the formation and retrieval of memories.

Bodyweight training also shows results in strength and size gains. One 2016 study[6] published in *Physiology & Behavior* investigated the amount of hypertrophy—the volume increase in tissue—over eighteen sessions of loaded and unloaded resistance training. Both formats showed similar gains, though the loaded movement group achieved greater improvements in muscle endurance.

As I said, size matters, and going all-out is a weightlifting trait. In lifting terminology, the focus is on continuing until you experience failure, doing as many reps as possible until your muscles literally cannot do another rep. While not necessarily bad, it can be exhausting, leading to overtraining—recovery is crucial. Before we get into our own bodyweight routine, let's explore failure as a mental state, for it offers profound insights into human psychology.

FAILING WELL

In weightlifting, failure is often a goal. Lift this amount of weight until your body crumbles. Maximum repetition becomes your benchmark. The failure mentality is declining with the recognition that pushing it to the max sometimes leads to breakdowns and injuries.[7] That said, the relationship between resistance and failure has an important psychological component.

Failure is not championed like success. Flip through the endless string of self-help, diet, and performance books. They promise success. Even this one is attempting to help you live optimally. I recognize that. This occurs for the same reason most Hollywood blockbusters don't end with the hero losing the girl (or guy, as Hollywood is catching up). If destiny were not achieved we wouldn't pay the entrance fee. We like to think we're the hero of our story. Humans are eternally optimistic. Yet we should not disavow the necessity of failure or try to pretend it's something other than it is. Failure is a valuable ally. As the Japanese proverb goes: fall down nine times, get up ten.

Failure has recently been lauded in Silicon Valley, where tech companies pay employees to pursue personal projects, many of which will lead nowhere. Some even create wings dedicated to thinking and experimenting. This flies counter to our risk-averse brains, which weigh losses with greater gravity than wins. The pleasure received from success is fleeting. We've often forgotten about it the next day in our pursuit of another goal. By contrast, the emotional damage of failure can last a lifetime. That's a shame, as we can use the frustration and uncertainty of failure to keep pushing forward.

British economist and journalist Tim Harford writes that there are three essential steps in using failure to your advantage: try new things, with the realization that some will fail; make sure that if you fail you will still survive—don't fail *too* big; know when you fail or you'll never learn.[8] Learning from failure is the pertinent point.

Psychology professor Carol Dweck is famous for her insights into fixed and growth mindsets.[9] As an example, she uses Michael Jordan as a growth mindset. After Jordan returned from his brief stint in baseball, the Chicago Bulls lost in the playoffs. Jordan was trying to live from past victories. During the off-season he learned a valuable lesson. His team then won three straight NBA championships. Dweck compares this to another elite athlete, John McEnroe, who lost in mixed doubles at Wimbledon in 1979. McEnroe hated losing—failing, in his mind—so much that he refused to play mixed doubles for twenty years. What could have been a teachable moment, in which he could have watched tapes of his performance and contemplated his swing, how he attacked the net, and how he interacted with his partner, instead turned into two decades of regret.

Failure opens up the pathway to creativity. The pressure of success is one of the surest methods of denying yourself pleasure in accomplishment. If you're incessantly craving an achievement yet feel losing is too big a burden to bear, you won't take any risks. I see this happen all the time in the gym: people remain embedded in their comfort zone. They don't attend the yoga class they know they should because they're afraid they can't do the postures correctly. They stay out of studio cycling because they don't have the proper shoes. That HIIT class looks too intense; they'll never look like the person in the front row. And so on.

We train our muscles with resistance to make them stronger. We learn our boundaries by failing. Once we find our edges we can grow beyond them. As in our muscles, so too in our brains, as another

Dweck study shows. During this study, which took place over the course of two years, Dweck had monitored students entering junior high school.[10] She removed over four hundred children from a dozen New York City schools after a test to praise each with a single sentence. Half of the students were told how intelligent they were. The other half were told they tried really hard. Intelligence, she knew, is a product of the fixed mindset: if you're smart, you're smart. Game over. These are the people who head straight to the treadmill every single gym visit, or the weight machines they know and love. Telling a student they tried hard implies there's room for growth. Plasticity. You did well this time, so you can do even better next. This, of course, is the chef with tight shoulders getting over her fears of inadequacy to enter the yoga studio because she knows that her career and life will benefit by loosening up. She goes in to fail so that she can succeed.

In fact, that is exactly what Dweck found. After the initial test she offered both groups the opportunity to take another. One was of equal challenge; the other was harder. Incredibly, of the group that she praised for effort, up to 90 percent chose the more challenging test. A majority of the intelligent students decided not to press their luck and chose the safe route. As she writes, they "went for the task that would allow them to keep on looking smart."[11]

When I was a child I was told I could be anything I wanted to be in life. Mine was not an isolated incident. This hopeful promise is part of our cultural ethos: try hard and succeed. What isn't discussed is how to fail. Like success, failure is an art. Some people do it well, while others run from any sign of it. They *resist* it. As we know from weightlifting, resistance is exactly what we want. Fail smart; fail often. Just don't fail too hard, as Harford warned. With that, let's build some muscle.

THE PROGRAM: RESISTANCE TRAINING

This section predominantly discussed studies on resistance training with weights, but that is only one form. As this is a bodyweight book designed for you to get strong and flexible anywhere, you'll only need your body.

Exercise #1: Jump and Fly

This movement combines two of my favorite strengthening exercises: tuck jumps and burpees with push-ups. While you can move quickly through these, remember the focus here is on strength. I recommend taking the push-up portion slower, adding explosive power in the tuck jump if you desire.

If you are jumping into your burpees, make sure your shoulders stay above your wrists as you jump back. I consistently witness students and clients allowing their body weight to pull their body back with their legs so they land with their shoulders inches behind their wrists. And if you are jumping, land with your elbows bent. Do not land in a high push-up (plank) position. Over time this will cause damage to your shoulders. If you want to begin in a plank, step back instead of jumping.

1. Begin with your feet shoulder distance apart. Squat slightly to generate power for the jump.
2. To perform a tuck jump, jump and bring your knees toward your chest. Keep your chest lifted during your ascent. If possible, land in a full squat. If you are not able to jump, simply perform a bodyweight squat instead of the jump.
3. From your squat, bring your hands down under your shoulders. Jump your legs back into a low push-up position. Slowly press back up. Keep your weight over your hands as you jump back into a squatting position.
4. If you are unable to jump back into a low-push up position, step back into a high push-up (plank), perform the push-up, then step or jump forward into a squat.
5. Repeat ten times. As you gain strength, lengthen it to twenty repetitions. Try not to stop the entire time. You don't have to go fast, but consistency is key.

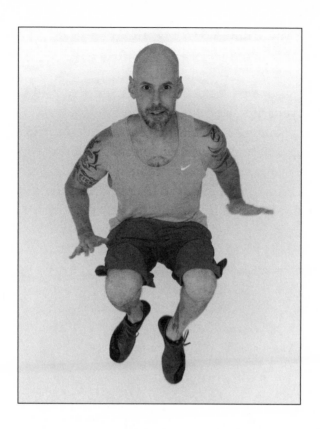

Exercise #2: Loaded Push-Ups

This movement covers your entire body: loaded beast gets into your ankle, knee, and hip joints, while the push-up works your entire body and core. To me this is the perfect example of training both flexibility and strength simultaneously.

1. Begin on your hands and knees with your shoulders directly above your wrists and hips above your knees. Tuck your toes. Lift your knees two inches from the ground.
2. Press your hips back toward your heels, as in a child's pose, with your knees hovering off the ground. This is loaded beast, as if you're about to explode forward into a run, if you were a four-legged creature. Actually, you are.

3. Bring your entire body forward into a plank position. Press back through your heels as your shoulders align over your wrists.
4. Perform one push-up. As soon as you return to your plank, press your hips back into loaded beast.
5. Ten repetitions to begin. Increase a little each week to keep seeing gains in strength and range of motion.

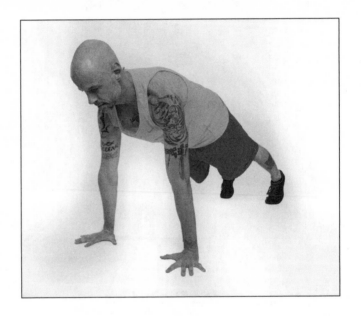

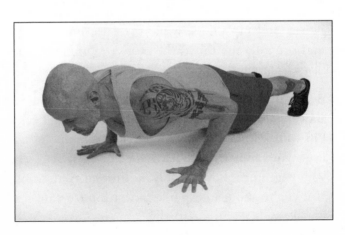

Exercise #3: Floating Sweeps

In the Brazilian martial art capoeira, a *negativa* is a low to the ground denial that blocks an offender. In this version, we'll jump from side to side, working in core and upper body strength while creating lower body mobility.

1. Begin in a fan posture (straddle forward bend) with your feet about three feet apart and your hands on the ground.
2. Rotate your left foot ninety degrees. Kick your right foot straight through to the left, hovering a few inches from the ground. Your weight is in your right arm, with the shoulder positioned directly above your wrist, as in a side plank posture.
3. As you return to the starting position, bring both hands to the ground, jump up into a pike position, and land with your right foot on the ground and your left leg extended out as in a kick.
4. As a modification, return to the fan posture each time before transitioning to the other side. Focus on alignment: shoulder above wrist, bent knee above ankle, kicking foot in flexion. If you're piking between sides, draw your knees in as you jump. More experienced practitioners can handstand between sides.

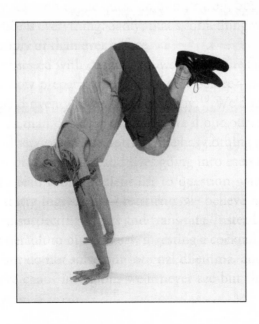

5. Perform six kicks on each side, and see if you can add another one (on each side) each week that you practice.

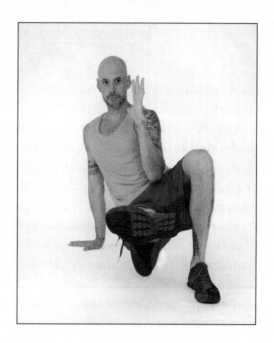

EXERCISE #4: PIKE UPS

While you may have performed a pike while jumping in the last exercise, this time you're going to pike your plank. This movement has it all: upper body and core strength, hip and shoulder flexibility. The slower you do this one, the better. Linger in the positions for a few breaths if you'd like. This is a great warm-up for all sorts of movements, or a wonderful stand-alone exercise.

1. Come into a plank posture with your shoulders directly above your wrists. Pike your plank by lifting your sitting bones toward the ceiling as you would in a downward facing dog. The key here it to engage your abdominal muscles while piking. If possible, bring your body weight forward more so that your shoulders are an inch or two in front of your wrists. The further forward you come, the harder it is to maintain.

2. Slowly exhale and let your hips sink toward the ground. Slide your feet back and roll over to the top of your feet. You'll finish in an upward facing dog, your shoulders directly above your wrists, your knees hovering off the ground, and your legs in isometric forward contraction to support the backbending position. Draw your shoulders down your back, move your sternum forward, and look straight ahead. Inhale.

3. On your exhale you'll return to the piking plank by engaging your abdominal muscles, as if someone were pressing lightly into them for the entire journey back. Try to roll over your feet to return them into a planking position. (I'm a huge fan of rolling over my feet to help with foot and ankle flexibility and mobility.)

4. Focus on maintaining proper shoulder position. Your hips and legs will drive this movement, supported by a strong commitment from your arms and upper body. The more your shoulders are in the proper position, the more challenging these will be, and the more you'll get out of it.

5. Perform ten. That's a lot if you're doing them slowly and properly, with one breath for each movement. Increase as you will, you beast.

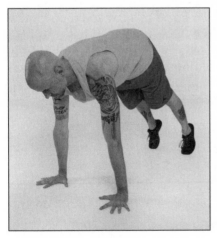 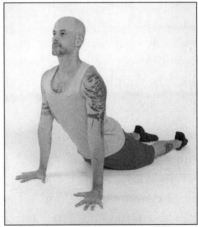

Chapter 7

Strike a Pose

"If the word 'yoga' *means* many things, that is because Yoga *is* many things."

—Mircea Eliade, *Yoga: Immortality and Freedom*

A PERFECT ANTIDOTE

When confronted with potential danger, your body freezes in preparation for battling, running, or to continue standing there, dumbfounded. Your adrenal medulla quickly secretes norepinephrine and epinephrine, the first preparing you for action by increasing blood flow to your muscles and output from your heart, the latter binding with liver cells to rapidly produce glucose for energy. Your amygdala, the brain's fear center, sets off your hypothalamus and pituitary gland, flooding you with ACTH (adrenocorticotropic hormone), which subsequently increases production of another stress hormone, cortisol. If struck, your blood clots more easily. Meanwhile, your white blood cells cling to the walls of your capillaries in case they need to fight off an infection. This cascade of chemicals accelerates your heart and breathing rates, slows your digestion, and frees up fat and glycogen for immediate energy—all markers of fighting. For those who freeze under stress, other effects—auditory impairment; tunnel vision; lost sphincter control—are destabilizing. Your body is in full stress mode.

Stress is necessary for survival and, as mentioned earlier, can sometimes be coopted for positive gains. While being on constant alert is unhealthy, this physiological response system serves humans in times of attack, whether by other tribes, animals, or errant weather patterns. Being ready at a moment's notice is required of those without walls, fences, and security systems. While our problems today are vastly different than millennia ago, we're still operating with the same internal hardware running the same basic software. Finding the balance between preparation and relaxation is essential for maintaining health. This is the space in which yoga enters.

As the Romanian scholar Mircea Eliade wrote (see above), yoga has meant many things during its slow evolution. Importantly, yoga is always a response to the environment. For ascetics it means retreating to a cave to grapple with their minds. For the oppressed it has served as a revolutionary political tool; bands of Indian warriors used yogic exercises in preparation for battling the British soldiers and merchants that were pillaging their land. For Indian nationalists at the turn of the twentieth century, yoga was a training sport that helped create strong bodies and minds in the fight for political independence. None of these are right or wrong; yoga's effects on your nervous system do not require any particular beliefs or affiliations. Yoga serves a function dependent upon when, where, and how it is practiced. Since such a discussion would require volumes, we're going to focus on the regenerative aspects of yoga, especially as it pertains to loosening your mental and emotional burdens, which I feel is why it's become so popular in modern societies.

As with resistance training, yoga works not by decreasing stress, but by increasing it temporarily. (Of course this depends on style: physically rigorous formats like Vinyasa and Ashtanga work in this manner; Nidra dives into parasympathetic mode from the start.) Yoga is a unique format in that it's both active and regenerative, often in the same class. In this book we began our journey slowly and will end on an equally chill note. Over the last two chapters the intensity level was raised. Yoga is the junction in which effort and effortlessness unite, though be warned, a dynamic salutation set like you're going to be practicing in a few pages may at first feel strenuous.

As yoga has soared in popularity over the past thirty years, many previous unaffiliated philosophies have attached itself to it. Outsiders treat it with derision, while advocates believe yoga is a panacea for every problem encountered in life. Naysayers claim it's "just stretching," a sentiment they often denounce once they've actually tried it. Yogis can become fundamentalist to their particular style as well as yoga in general. None of these attitudes are helpful. Before we dive into yoga's health benefits we'll briefly discuss its origins to better understand the intentions behind this beautiful discipline.

MAN WITH A VISION

We'll probably never know the actual origins of yoga. The earliest evidence of anything related to yoga dates back to 3000 BC in the Indus Valley region. Archaeological excavations at Mohenjo-daro and Harappa (both in present-day Pakistan) uncovered earthenware seals depicting a man seated cross-legged surrounded by animals.[1] Given that this mythological symbolism is related to Shiva, the god of yoga, the coins became known as "proto-Shiva."

Fast forward two millennia as *kriyas* appear in Indian texts. These were purification rituals that mainly involved intense breathing exercises. Yoga did not arrive to modernity whole cloth, but was eventually compiled roughly 1,600 years ago by an unknown man named Patanjali in *Yoga Sutra*. *Sutra* means thread (related to "suture"); Patanjali wove together ideas from six different philosophical systems. The term "yoga" was initially used devotionally: bhakti yoga, most famously known from the classic text, *Bhagavad Gita*, is the teaching of an incarnation of the god Krishna instructing the young archer, Arjuna. Born into the warrior caste, Arjuna is in the midst of an existential crisis; he is called to kill friends and cousins on the battlefield. Krishna basically tells him to man up, reminding Arjuna that as a man born into the warrior caste his duty is to destroy. So much for the peaceful origins of yoga.

Strangely, this does in some ways mimic what we now practice. Arjuna's dilemma causes him anxiety. Instead of calming the bowman through meditation or avoiding the situation completely, Krishna instructs him to move into discomfort. Only then will he emerge a wiser man. He settles into his stress, which is *exactly* what we're training our body and mind to do today, no bows required.

While recent research[2] has shown that Patanjali's masterwork has only recently become influential, *Yoga Sutra* offers many insights. Eliade was one of the first modern scholars to seriously undertake an academic study of this Indian art. Using Patanjali as a guide, Eliade views yoga as a means of self-analysis. In fact, Eliade believed ancient yogis were doing more beneficial work than the burgeoning field of psychiatry. As he writes, "knowledge of the systems of 'conditioning' could not be an end in itself; it was not knowing them that mattered, but mastering them."[3] In this sense conditioning means recognizing mental patterns. Bringing your issues to light is just the beginning. The varied techniques involved in "burning" them—fire is often employed as a metaphor—through spirited yogic rituals is the critical next step. These include rapid breathing (something we should reconsider, as it over-stimulates your nervous system while cutting off oxygen to your brain), twisting your body into contorted shapes, and spending hours in focused meditation. While yoga today is generally gentler (albeit more aerobic and strength-building), the goal is similar: coming to terms with your inner anxieties and—this is key—recognizing that your body is an integral part of this process, something psychoanalysis often misses, as Eliade observed. Freedom from internal chatter requires physicality as well as mental fortitude and emotional endurance. By tuning into your body, your ability to focus strengthens.

Yoga took its modern form at the turn of the twentieth century as part of a nationalistic movement spurred by Indians seeking independence from British colonialism. A strong body and mind were equated to a strong will. To compete with a growing culture of weight lifting and gymnastics, a young man from the region of Karnataka named Tirumalai Krishnamacharya reinvented yoga into what we know today.[4] All modern lineages in some way trace back to him. Borrowing from wrestling, gymnastics, and bodybuilding, Krishnamacharya made yoga more physical than ever before.

Americans were not ignorant of yoga during this time. They had discovered it a century prior, mostly through efforts by Ralph Waldo Emerson and the Theosophical movement. As the world became smaller, Americans tapped into an expanding well of yoga *asanas* (postures) for health and show. Yoga might have originated with meditation and moral questions, but our visual system seeks attention. Pictures of a shirtless Theos Barnard circulating in the thirties offered new means for getting healthy. While yoga would not infiltrate the mainstream for another sixty years, today it is a $16 billion dollar industry boasting thirty-six million adherents in America alone.[5]

Part of Krishnamacharya's genius was in modifying yoga for the population he taught. While working with older clients with nagging injuries he developed a slower, methodical style that addressed their individual bodies. One of Krishnamacharya's main students (and brother-in-law), B. K. S. Iyengar, tutored under him, which is how Iyengar Yoga developed. Later in his life Krishnamacharya was assigned to teach a group of young boys. He knew that a slow, exacting style would never calm the little demons down, so he invented a vigorous, flowing series of postures that another student, Pattabhi Jois, borrowed from when creating Ashtanga Yoga. Viniyoga and Sai Yoga also developed out of Krishnamacharya's teachings. In his hands, yoga morphed and evolved through a number of phases, though each kept the "union" (the etymological root of "yoga") of body and mind intact. Today, there are thousands of adjectives preceding the noun "yoga" to differentiate one teacher's approach over others. At the heart of it all, however, is this union. If it is lost, so is yoga. Then, it really is "just stretching."

INTO THE FIRE

Not that stretching is bad. I'll take it over a lack of stretching any day. Yoga requires the participant to deliberately shift awareness into the present moment. Stretching while texting does not result in yoga; how well you're stretching at that point is also up for debate. Whether you're flowing through a series of sun salutations breath by breath or holding each posture for minutes at a time, the focused direction of your cognitive resources is the primary aim. While a ton of hearsay exists regarding the extent of benefits, a number of studies have detailed yoga's credibility.

Let's start with stress reduction. A healthy body coming down from fight-flight-freeze mode flips the switch to activate parasympathetic mode. The problem is that many of us remain on high alert, whether due to excessive doses of caffeine or an addiction to smartphones. While I'm a big fan of technology, being on alert 24/7 can cripple your nervous system. Yoga is an antidote to constantly itching for a text ding, which is why I discourage students from having their phone next to their mats. While there are reasonable circumstances for doing this, such as doctors on call or parents with children, most often phones serve as reminders of moments outside of the studio. Texting up until the moment of the first posture only to rush back to it the second that the *Savasana* (corpse pose) ends is not a healthy way to approach yoga. Or anything, really.

Stress is considered the world's leading killer for its role in either directly causing or helping promote heart disease, obesity, type 2 diabetes, depression, strokes, and osteoporosis. While stress does not appear to cause cancer, it certainly doesn't help after the crippling effects of chemotherapy or radiation. Anxiety also reduces levels of BDNF production, stunting the ability to retain information.[6] The obesity connection is especially stark in children; elevated cortisol levels make them hungrier. To combat stressful emotions they often turn to comfort foods that are predominantly rich in carbohydrates and sugar. Elevated cortisol increases triglyceride levels, systolic and diastolic blood pressure, insulin resistance, and fasting blood sugar. It's not only the quality of food spurring obesity; cortisol specifically causes your body to store visceral fat in your abdomen. Add to the list poor sleep, mood swings, memory problems, increased inflammation, and chronic fatigue, and you understand how stress is such a potent and encompassing killer.

One mechanism in which yoga reduces anxiety is by increasing the brain's GABA (gamma-Aminobutyric acid) levels. GABA is an inhibitory neurotransmitter that exhibits an anti-anxiety effect by reducing neuronal excitability. One study found that yogis experienced a 27 percent increase in GABA levels (the non-yoga group showed a zero-percent increase); one experienced yogi in the group displayed a 47 percent rise, while another, who practices five times a week, reached 80 percent.[7] Another study found yoga more effective than walking in terms of increasing GABA levels.[8]

From a neurobiological perspective, yoga initiates a conversation between your limbic system, where emotions begin, and your rational prefrontal cortex. This is where focus (or, as many instructors state, intention) comes into play. Remember, if your attention is completely absorbed with how much you're struggling and how intense the limb contortions are, you'll remain in sympathetic mode. It doesn't have to be this way. Techniques such as deepening your breath, softening your forehead, and shifting your mental focus change your relationship to your body. The discomfort and disorientation experienced during a class can be reframed by shifting your attention to the quality of your breath or the positive sensations of working out.[9] This is again similar to Kelly McGonigal's advice of reframing stress as an energetic resource. Intention matters.

Most yoga is practiced in studios surrounded by like-minded individuals. You're (hopefully) in a safe space. A smart instructor keeps drawing your attention to relaxing into the poses rather than fighting against them. I've found this especially difficult to express to men, who are accustomed to sports and workouts that require immense power and strength; strength in yoga is soft and fluid. Smooth, controlled breathing moves you into parasympathetic mode, shifting your body away from the stress response. Even though you're in a demanding situation, your nervous system is not overwhelmed. You're training your brain to not invoke the stress response even though the situation you are in is stressful. This is one powerful way to take yoga "off the mat."

Isn't this old folk wisdom? Take a deep breath? Yes, though the effects don't stop there. Yoga is a comprehensive exercise. The physiological slowdown reduces stress, heart rate, and blood pressure while boosting immunity response and reducing hypertension. Yoga has also been shown to raise levels of antioxidants and lower oxidative stress in blood, improve balance (especially important for seniors), and counteract deterioration in vertebral disks. These regenerative effects help in the maintenance of your body and mind. They also keep you limber and flexible for whatever other workouts are ahead.

One of the most touted benefits in yoga is weight loss, which it accomplishes in a roundabout way. Remember, yoga is a response to an environment, and Americans struggle with weight. It's not as simple as doing a thousand boat poses to "strengthen your core." The minimal aerobic effects (yoga is not an aerobic exercise) aren't going to "burn away tummy fat." Those are sales gimmicks by shifty instructors. Reducing cortisol levels *can* help you reduce visceral fat, however. This is counterintuitive to how yoga is presented: it's not the sweat and hustle but the calm and collected state of mind that leads to potential weight loss. There's also nothing wrong with throwing Pilates into the mix. That will firm things up, but has little to do with actual fat deposits. That's better addressed through nutrition.

Science is built through research and verification. Most of what we hear about is quantitative results: this measured that, that percentage of people does it like this. Then there's qualitative research, which relies on anecdotes. While you and I might feel very different after the same yoga session, time and again yoga studies reveal that people feel better about themselves after class. How we feel about ourselves impacts how we view the world. For example, yoga has measurably been shown to improve executive functioning, which means we're able to inhibit negative emotional responses and increase working memory. This positively alters how we feel about ourselves. Other research has shown yoga helps us self-regulate, foster attention and concentration, reduce aggression, and increase body awareness, examples of what research literature calls positive psychological empowerment.

As stress is minimized you function better. Yet this basic physiological fact seems unrecognizable in the chaos of daily life: bills, road rage, politics, an entire landscape of potential threats and emotional danger. Disengaging from society—not voting; remaining unconcerned about environmental catastrophes; being selfish—is not the answer. I'm an advocate for balance at every level of society. Yoga is a wonderful means for finding balance somewhere between looking inward and expressing outward.

I generally hear two responses from people that do not practice yoga: *I'm Type A* and *I'm not flexible*. The irony, of course, is that yoga addresses both. For the obsessive and compulsive, it offers tools to alleviate the constant mental chatter by bringing the object of attention into focus. This will be discussed more in the next chapter on meditation, which is complementary to this discussion. As for flexibility, you're never going to become flexible by *not* stretching. The insistence that oneself is not flexible is usually indicative of someone who feels self-conscious in a group setting, which is one reason online yoga instruction is so popular. If that is you, recognize that if someone in class is judging you, that's their problem, not yours. Easier said than done, sure, but reframing how you approach your body is important for growth. Attitude and physicality are tightly linked. The discomfort of showing up is worthwhile.

Besides, stretching feels good. Inflexibility is inattention. If you can't hold a stretch for a sustained period of time, it's going to be challenging to witness actual structural change in your joints. (While we usually envision muscles when discussing flexibility, the term is defined as an ability to move your joints through a wide range of motion. Obviously muscle tension plays a role in this.) This is different from dynamic stretching, which in yoga means moving through postures, such as sun salutations or an interval of squats, which also increase your range of motion. In certain forms of yoga, such as Hatha and Bikram, postures are held for a sustained period, while in Vinyasa ("flowing with breath") you're transitioning from pose to pose more rigorously. I prefer and teach classes that include sustained (or static) and dynamic stretching. To be clear, there are other forms of stretching, including ballistic, which includes bouncing movements (rarely used in yoga); active isolated stretching, a rehabilitative form in which you move through a specific sequence without holding any portion for more than two seconds (most often used in yoga with a strap while sitting or lying on the floor); and proprioceptive neuromuscular facilitation, which requires another person.

Since static and dynamic stretching is predominant in yoga, we'll focus on those.

In sports, dynamic stretching involves mimicking the movements you're going to do in the activity itself. Translating to yoga, runners are well served with lunges, while basketball players want to focus on squats and twists, as well as calf and foot stretches to aid in the explosive power needed for the sport. Dynamic stretching should be done before any sport, static stretching during recovery. This is because dynamic stretches do not improve tissue extensibility, while static stretches do. If you're going for a run the last thing you want is to have just held long stretches. Given the impact force your body is about to take, your muscles want to be warm but not deformed. After a trail run, this is exactly what you want, however—a little after the run, that is, and then regularly in recovery.

Knowing when and how to stretch involves rethinking your movement patterns. Do you always put on one pant leg before the other? Tie a particular shoe first? How about getting up from a chair? Do you press into your feet to stand, or put your left hand on the chair's arm to push up? What about walking: does your right foot turn out a bit more than the left? For the most part we all have the same basic parts. How we move about the world influences our gait, posture, and even attitude. Consider this: how is Sisyphus, the deceitful prince who was punished by having to push a boulder up a hill that would inevitably roll back down, portrayed? Shoulders rounded, sternum caved, chin jutting, head hung low. Very much like modern office workers, in fact. Now consider the accommodating metaphor: carrying the weight of the world on your back. If you're always slouched forward at your computer or gazing at your phone, your posture suffers, the quality of your thinking suffers, everything suffers.

Now picture people we call strong: chest lifted, head upright, chin held high, eyes straight ahead or slightly into the distance. Uprightness comes with great sociological benefits as unconscious mechanisms of perception greatly influence cultures. Standing up tall and facing the world is universally regarded, while shirking from responsibility is a sign of weakness and uncertainty. Poor sitting and texting habits play into this, as does consistently weight training and running without countering the deformities of those workouts with opposing actions.

The point is our physical actions need to be balanced. Take two of the most important: pushing and pulling. In yoga there is a lot of pushing. In plank you're pushing; lower to *Chaturanga*, the low push-up position. Still pushing. Is the next posture in the traditional sequence, upward facing dog, an example of pulling? No. You need an external force or load to pull. To counteract the constant pushing you need to do pull-ups or other forms of resistance training, such as rows. Yogis overtrain one aspect of essential movement. If they don't ever pull, balance will be impossible.

If you're pushing all the time, like weightlifters obsessively focused on chest muscles, and never reverse with shoulder and pectoral stretches, you have a whole different set of problems to contend with. Rounded shoulders create a forward head tilt, which beyond adding stress to your neck muscles also affects your vestibular system, which is responsible for balance. This position creates an anterior pelvic tilt, inviting a range of lower and middle back issues. One of the most common problems I address with students and clients is a tight quadratus lumborum (QL) muscle, which connects your pelvis to your spine. This muscle is often overtrained and understretched (or under-massaged). It is also one of the most common sources of lower back pain.

This muscle in particular is a good example of why pre-workout dynamic stretching and post-workout static stretching are essential. Lack of stretching increases tissue viscosity, leading to chronic damage. Most of our body is a combination of elasticity and plasticity. With light loads we have a greater range of motion; with heavier loads, we respond by tightening up to protect tissues, muscles, and joints from potential damage. When you lose flexibility you're more susceptible to injuries and back pain. You're more plastic than elastic. You want to be strong, but you also want to be pliable.

Yoga is the perfect cross-training tool with an endless array of benefits that exceed simply countering the effects of intense workouts and daily movement patterns. I've intentionally left out the philosophical background of yoga; this is addressed in a previous book if you are interested.[10] I'll be discussing more of the neurological benefits of yoga in the next chapter. For now let's focus on stretching. Designing a personal practice that specifically addresses your personal needs will not only help you feel better physically, but also it will help you perform in all aspects of life. In general, use your body as a guide. Don't avoid tight or weak spots; they don't improve when you pretend they don't exist. The patience you learn spending time focused during these stretches translates into your mental and emotional worlds as well. More on that soon. For now let's get on the mat.

THE PROGRAM: YOGA

Exercise #1: Flow with It

This Vinyasa yoga sequence consists of twelve postures linked together to create a flow. I suggest flowing through this three times on each side. On the first two rounds, flow through one breath per movement. On the third round, hold each posture for five breaths. While I'm writing the explanations below, visit wholemotion.com to view the flow in action, which will give you a better sense of how to transition between postures and where the alignment points are.

1. Begin in downward facing dog. Spread out your fingers slightly and find a firm foundation with your entire hands pressing into the floor.
2. Step your right foot into a low lunge. Lower your left knee to the ground (slide a towel or blanket underneath if needed, or, if you have any knee issues, keep it lifted). Lift your arms up toward the ceiling, keeping your shoulder blades drawing down your back.

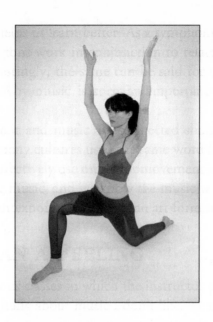

3. Release both hands inside of your right foot. Allow your right knee to open away from your body into a pigeon lunge. Press your right hand into your right thigh, gently twisting from your midsection toward the ceiling. Do your best to not allow your left hip to twist; keep that hip parallel to the floor. Draw your right shoulder blade toward your spine as you gently press your right leg open.

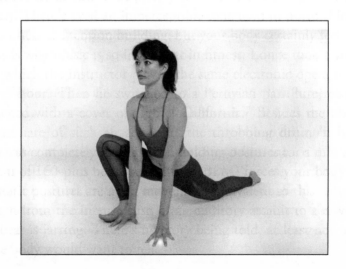

4. With your left shoulder above your left wrist, raise your right arm to the ceiling. Slowly straighten both legs into a rotational side plank pose. You'll be on the outer edges of both feet, so that the left side of your body is in a traditional side plank, while your right foot remains where it was. Keep your left shoulder above your left wrist as you lift your hips up and back. Don't force your right leg to straighten completely.

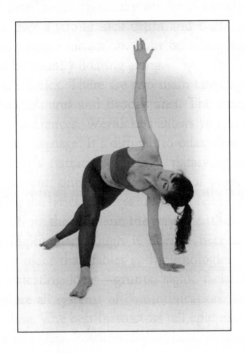

5. Come out of the twist and rotate both feet back to the ground. Lower both forearms inside of your right foot into lizard pose. (Slide a block under your forearms if necessary.) Your right toes are pointing forward with your right knee directly above your right foot. Your back knee can remain on the ground, or tuck your left toes and extend through that leg for more stretch. Notice if there's more weight on your left forearm than your right. If so you can angle your upper body to the left slightly to spread out the weight on your forearms. Pull your sternum toward your thumbs to take any roundedness out of your upper back.

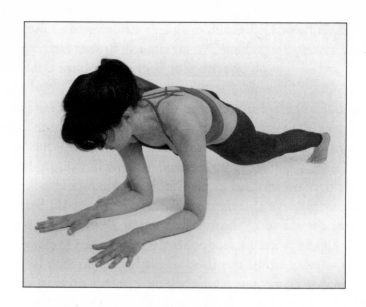

6. Lower your left knee if it's lifted. Walk back onto your hands, then straighten your right leg and fold over it into a runner's lunge. You can keep your hips above your left knee or sit all the way back onto your left heel, which will add an ankle stretch.

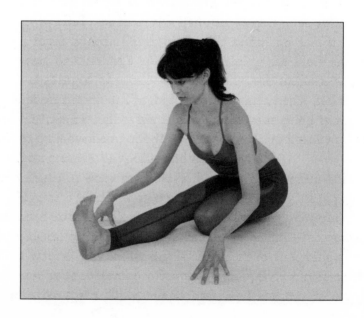

7. Bending your right knee, tuck your left toes and shift into a curtsy lunge, with your left knee behind your right calf muscles, your arms extended behind you, and your torso lifted.

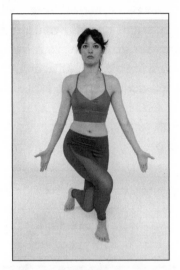

8. Press into your right foot and slowly lift your back leg into a Warrior Three pose. With your left foot flexed, extend that leg to the wall behind you in this balancing position. Choose where to bring your arms: behind you by your sides, palms together in front of your sternum, or arms extended to the wall in front of you.

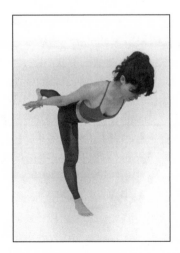

9. Bending your right knee, step back into Warrior One. Reach your arms toward the ceiling with your shoulder blades drawing down your back. Imagine you're holding a block between your hands to create isometric engagement in your upper back. Make sure your right knee is bending directly over your right foot, with the outside edge of your back foot pressed into the floor. (For those of you with knee or ankle injuries, rotate your back heel up so you're in a high lunge.)

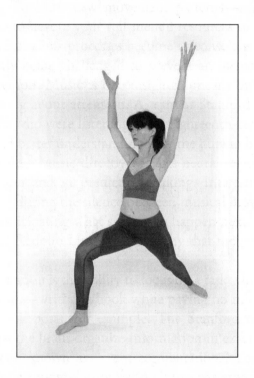

10. Interlace your hands behind your lower back, extending your forearms away from your sacrum. Broadening through your collarbones, bring your torso forward inside of your right thigh for devotional warrior. Maintain neutral hip alignment from Warrior One as you fold. Your outer left hip will continue to square forward, with your right sit bones drawing toward the back wall.

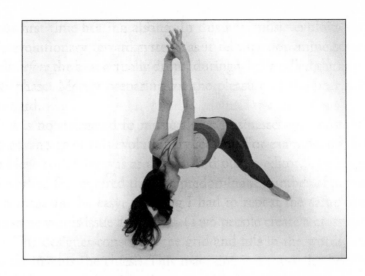

11. Pressing into your left foot, lift your torso to Reverse Warrior. Bring your left hand to your back thigh and extend your right arm toward the back wall, drawing your right shoulder blade down your back.

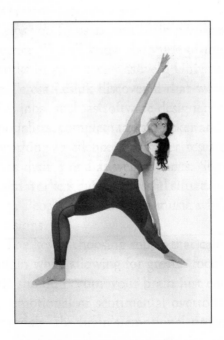

12. Slowly bend your left leg into side lunge. Place your left hand down and extend your right arm up into a twist toward the front of your mat. Make sure that your left heel stays grounded and your left knee lines up right over the middle of your left foot. As a modification bring both hands onto the floor and gently ease your hips back. The goal is not to get as low as possible. Once you feel the rotational thigh stretch, you've gone far enough.

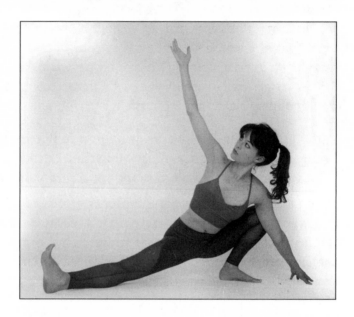

13. Rotate toward the front of your mat, stepping back into downward facing dog, or flowing to low push up, upward facing dog, and back to downward dog. Take one breath, then repeat on your left side. On your third round take five breaths in each posture.

Chapter 8

Tuning In

"If we commit ourselves to staying right where we are, then our experiences become very vivid. Things become very clear when there is nowhere to escape."

—Pema Chödrön, *When Things Fall Apart*

THE MIRACLE OF CHEMISTRY

What a long, strange journey meditation has taken. When I was first introduced to it in the mid-nineties, meditation was still for the crunchy and hippie, even though various styles had been embedded in American social circles for centuries. Naysayers assume navel-gazing means inactivity, an excuse for not confronting the hard realities of the actual world. If only they knew the tremendous work it takes to slow down the incessant churnings of one's mind, as well as how much *that* world influences the *real* one. If thinking is internalized movement, our mind is not one to stop moving— meditation is not, it should be noted, about stopping your thoughts. Simply trying to control what and how you think requires tremendous effort, but the benefits of this process are immense.

Though Americans gazed askew at meditators for generations, somewhere along the way it caught on. Today it's impossible to miss another CEO or superstar athlete touting meditation's miraculous benefits. As with other workouts in this book, the miracle is chemical. If you don't consider meditation a workout, perhaps we need to redefine the term, for nothing is as daunting as focusing on focusing. You might not sweat, but you will be tried. Meditation is the epitome of the brain challenging itself.

Visually, meditation is often presented seated, legs crossed, eyes closed, in deep contemplation. While this is certainly one way to approach it, the original definition of the term is to think something over or "considering something thoughtfully."[1] When something weighs on our mind we meditate on it. In *The Symposium*, Plato discusses Socrates's incredible mental prowess. The great philosopher remained unfazed during a famine while in times of plenty he drank everyone under the table without becoming tipsy. Socrates proved equally unmatched in thought. He once stood still for an entire day and night mulling over a problem, unresponsive to anyone pestering him. His well-trained mind was unmovable yet supple, introspective while flexible.

As with yoga (in many ways, yoga and meditation are synonymous; postures developed as preparatory exercises for contemplation), meditation means many things to many people. For our purposes, let's define meditation as cultivating an ability to slow the barrage of thoughts in your mind in order to help you focus. There have been numerous other purported benefits, many of which might be true. We'll stay on track by first looking at the regenerative properties of meditation, then we'll explore why it's a powerful way to study the brain-body connection. After that, we'll sit, or stand, or walk, depending on how we want to experience the development of mindfulness.

As with yoga, people have often told me, "I'm no good at meditating" and "I'm too Type A to meditate." My response remains the same: you have to practice to reap the benefits. The literature confirms its value.

REGENERATION NATION

No figure has influenced our understanding of meditation as much as Richard J. Davidson. He became interested in it while studying psychology at Harvard, a secret he kept to himself, as academics were highly skeptical that anything could be achieved sitting around "doing nothing." Strange as it seems now, critics felt that emotion and cognition were separate domains, each playing no role in influencing the other. Davidson provided proof that they do when he mapped the neural pathways of emotion using an electroencephalogram (EEG).

Davidson traveled to India to study meditation while keeping his home practice under wraps. He knew sitting each day helped him cope with the rigors of academia. He just didn't know how to prove it. The development of EEG and fMRI technologies offered him the means, while a challenge by Tenzin Gyatso, the current Dalai Lama, afforded him the inspiration to commence with scientific research. Scanning the brains of seasoned meditators lit up his cortical maps. Novices registered at a lower frequency. Since then, decades of exploration have linked meditation with emotional states and, most importantly, shown that a focused practice helps you alter your emotional responses to stimulation. One of the first revelations, as longtime practitioners knew even if they couldn't pinpoint the physiological reason, was a reduction in anxiety.

We've established that a critical aspect of regeneration is stress relief. When you're not bogged down by the manifold anxieties of existence, your system functions more efficiently. Humans today have fewer problems than generations past, yet it's hard to come to terms with the fact that most of us are really lucky. We were born into a world of vaccines, technology, science, grocery stores, and advanced health care. I'm not glossing over the financial and political struggles many millions of people face every day. Even though I have not discussed the sociological aspects of fitness, they should certainly still be considered. Many people cannot afford gym memberships, which is, in part, why I wrote this book. Regardless of availabilities such as time, money, and equipment, we are *generally* better off than ever before. Everyone functions more optimally when less stressed. It's easier to be kind and compassionate, forgiving and charitable, when not bogged down with gripping crises echoing in our heads. If we can get those under control, a more receptive and peaceful state of mind extends outward to affect others. Humans learn best by example, so best to be a positive one.

Meditation is one training ground for the development of an empathic attitude. You're more caring of others when you take care of yourself. One issue some take with meditation is the long periods of time required. Yet even a brief training of only four days enhances an individual's ability to sustain attention while reducing fatigue and anxiety.[2] Further research found that mindfulness meditation helps alleviate sleep disturbances[3] and chronic pain,[4] both huge factors in performance. Controlling your mind effectively means having a say in how your nervous system responds to challenges. Meditation helps by activating the neural structures that control your autonomic nervous system, which governs unconscious bodily processes, such as heart rate, digestion, and breathing.[5] By having a say in these processes, you alleviate distress in your thinking. Put simply, when you feel good, you think and act better. You also heal faster, which concurrently aids you in growing stronger. Your immune system and mindset are interdependent.

Like yoga, meditation is a construct of and response to the culture practicing it. Altering consciousness has been pursued for millennia through a variety of means, including meditation, intense breathing exercises, rhythmic music, ritual theater, and hallucinogenic drugs. Just as each of these will produce different cognitive and physiological effects, how you meditate affects which brain regions are altered. For example, one study focused on the brain's beta, theta, and gamma activity through three different styles of meditation: open monitoring, focused attention, and automatic self-transcending.[6] The researchers found that each style had different effects.

Thus, treating meditation as a catchall term is misleading. Not every meditation style works for everyone; sometimes it takes a bit of work and patience to figure out what resonates with you. What's important is to stick to a regular practice and, perhaps counterintuitively, to quit while you're ahead. Buddhist scholar Robert Thurman believes that if you force yourself to sit for twenty minutes but peter out after five, you're going to dread practicing. Instead, sit for four, stop while you're having a pleasant experience, and you'll want to return the next day. When you associate pleasure with meditation you'll look forward to it, thereby increasing the time and effort you put into your practice.

As stated, benefits are immense. Meditation is more than a metaphor, as it actually changes the physical structures of your brain. The chemical reactions exhibit tangible correlations. Consider how we speak: *There's a pit in my stomach. I'm lighter than a feather. My blood is boiling. I feel so heavy. The weight of the world is on my shoulders.* Anxiety raises your blood pressure; it gets your blood boiling. Counter such sensations with contentedness, feeling good in your body. One of the results of contentedness is a stronger immune system. By feeling good about yourself, you're less likely than chronically unhappy people to get sick.[7] In fact, Richard Davidson conducted that particular experiment twice because he couldn't believe meditators had a better immune response and quicker healing times than the non-meditating group. But they did. Positive mental imagery regarding one's body and mental outlook increases levels of growth hormone, prolactin, and oxytocin. The first two bind to white blood cell receptors, which helps battle infection. Oxytocin decreases both blood pressure and cortisol levels.[8] Mindfulness meditation leads to quicker and more efficient regeneration of your cells.

Retraining your brain spans a number of fields. Another related course of action is behavioral activation therapy. Feeling positive about yourself is a chemical reaction strengthened by shifting your mental awareness. The nucleus accumbens sits near your hypothalamus. It plays many roles, including processing fear and encoding new motor patterns. It also helps you handle aversion, pleasure and reward, reinforcement, and motivation. Certain people who suffer from depression cannot sustain activity in their nucleus accumbens; positive emotions, such as those learned through the pleasure and reward process, quickly fade away. Like social groups, brain regions work together. When the nucleus accumbens is activated through pleasure, so is a region in your prefrontal cortex called the middle prefrontal gyrus, which contains numerous dopamine receptors. Depression seems to cause disconnect between these two regions; one speaks while the other refuses to listen. A 2009 study in depressed patients found that 75 percent showed a marked reduction in depression symptoms after twelve weeks of behavioral activation therapy[9], which is a method that promotes environmental reinforcement instead of punishment.

This is important, as meditation also reframes self-perception. Your brain's paralimbic system is referred to as your reptilian brain. Directly connected to your spinal cord, it controls your heart rate, breathing, balance, and internal temperature—autonomic functions involved in the fight-flight-freeze system. While it sits evolutionarily lower than your neocortex, the reasoning brain responsible for rational thought, imagination, abstract thought, and language, these two regions are intimately connected. People who have a difficult time controlling their emotions exhibit quick reaction signals from the paralimbic to the neocortex, as if they had no time to process what's happening before lashing out in fear or anger—because there *was no time*. They actually don't realize such a skill set is possible to develop.

This is a trained behavior. Genetics plays a role, as does environment. As I mentioned earlier, dualism—there is another me inside of me—is an outdated model of physiology. Yet it accounts for such an emotional response: *I have no control*, as if there's someone else operating your system. People who claim they have no control over their emotions are not necessarily being untruthful, but they are also victims of their own patterns. (Certain disorders *are* insurmountable without chemical intervention or, in the case of schizophrenics, not at all at the moment.) As we know from neuroplasticity, patterns can change. Meditation is one such agent.

While the term "spiritual" is often associated with practices like yoga and meditation, I'm hard put to think of anything deeper than having control over your emotions. How in charge of your reactions are you in response to stimulation? Can you control the flow of your thoughts, or do you feel victimized by them? If you're having a thought you don't enjoy, can you shift it quickly, or does it takes minutes, hours, days, weeks? Your identity is the product of your thought patterns; your history plays an integral role in defining your reality. We create a world inside of our heads based on experience. All experiences produce chemical reactions; that chemistry defines who you are.

Want to change that picture? Have a seat.

Just as how we process our experiences influences our identity, we need others to fully form a sense of self. Social connections are our great tool of triumph over the elements. When a society organizes harmoniously, everyone is taken care of; when resources are allocated only to a very few, discord reigns. Much the same occurs in our heads. Davidson termed the process by which the synchronous waves connect the brain regions "phase-locking," a state we want to achieve. The life around us might not cater to our every need, but our relationship to it shifts when our neural regions are in communication. Meditation helps phase-locking occur. A calm brain, he writes, is like a lake, while the "background cacophony" of unorganized noise creates in our lives a "turbulent sea."[10] Meditation is not the only tool that helps us phase-lock, but it is an important one.

Like the diverse nature of your social groups, variety in your movement and thought patterns helps you stay flexible and open to other possibilities. This is not just in relationship to your body. In fact, the body and brain junction is experienced in no greater detail than in meditation. You need a body to do it, but you are also drastically altering your neural patterns. That shifts everything physical, mental, and emotional. You emerge from your seat transformed. The more you return, the more the changes stick.

There are two meditations at the end of this chapter. Mindfulness is a general approach to tapping into the processes we've been discussing. Then there's a more specific style called *tonglen*, a Tibetan Buddhist meditation meaning "giving and taking." This one involves diving deeply into uncomfortable sensations. It is designed to help you give up attachments and be more loving, but the route is directly into the source of your pain. Feeling pain reminds you that you are a sentient being with consciousness, which is the final piece in the first half of our journey together. Consciousness is a word used so frequently as to be almost meaningless, yet it is also the vehicle that gives us meaning. It helps us give meaning to the world. The next half of the book is all about your mind, so best to know a little about the engine propelling it forward.

THE LITTLE ENGINE THAT COULD

Of all the terms in psychology, *metacognition* is my favorite: we know that we know. Like an aerial photographer, we look down at the timeline of our lives and guess the future, the long-term implication of Rodolfo Llinás's art of prediction. This ability to peer backward and forward is truly unique in the animal kingdom. It developed sometime over the last six million years since our common ancestor diverged from the chimpanzee line. Memory and foresight are such ingrained skills that we hardly imagine them novel. But they are. We lack many skills that other mammals possess. We're incredibly slow, stunningly weak, unnecessarily loud, and peculiarly egocentric. But we work well with others and can imagine a better future thanks to tools passed down through the generations. Even our close cousins, the Neanderthals, couldn't pull that off. They used the same stone technologies with no advancement for hundreds of thousands of years.[11] We're perturbed if a web page won't load in under two seconds.

How did we achieve this ability to know that we know, to step behind the curtain and become the great and powerful orchestrator of change? For much of this book I've discussed gaffes in thinking we're better than our environment, how we suffer mismatch diseases at every turn. Yet the more I study neuroscience, the more profoundly awed I am by the exquisite nature of consciousness. Our brains are the most complex organs known: ten trillion neurons with some one thousand trillion connections chatting inside a three-pound organ encased by our skull.[12] Still, the very term "consciousness" is murky and unsettled. Even experts can't agree as to what *it* is.

Most of us don't wake up contemplating ways to strengthen our brain. We don't obsess over its shape, whether it's too fat or not muscular enough. Yet this organ makes us obsess over our overall physical shape in such ways. All of our neurotic dispositions and dislikes, our pleasures and triumphs, originate with the relationship our nervous system has with our environment. This occurs thanks to the mechanism we call consciousness. Before beginning our meditation, let us consider what this entails. Remember, meditation implies thinking something over. What better than to contemplate the act of contemplation itself?

Let's churn these thoughts through the lens of yoga. Undoubtedly the most cited aphorism in Patanjali's *Yoga Sutra* is the second: *yogas-citta-vrtti-nirodah.* Although numerous translations of these four words exist, I'm partial to late scholar Georg Feuerstein: *Yoga is the restriction of the fluctuations of consciousness.*[13] Patanjali expounds those fluctuations in depth while prescribing techniques for their restriction. Slowing the neuronal firings that assault our brain with a ceaseless stream of thought is the goal of meditation. Numerous practices have been developed to address our mind chatter. While some are dedicated to transcending the physical body, we know the workings of our brain are embodied. The real challenge is developing a relationship with your brain where you control the fluctuations of thinking. While beautiful metaphors are expressed in scriptures like the *Sutra*, today we have more detail as to the chemical and physiological basis of consciousness. If we want to address the self, consciousness's great creation, we are better served studying the reality of our nervous system than the poetry of old.

The human brain is composed of a complex network of neurons communicating with one another by propagating an electrical current that travels along a tube-like channel called an axon. The current runs into another neuron at the tip, the synapse, causing the release of a chemical molecule, the transmitter. There are more potential neuronal connections in a single human brain than elementary particles in the entire universe. A neuron colliding with a muscle fiber, for example, results in movement. Thinking is literally a fluctuation, not just metaphorically. As we've established, thought is movement.

Our conception of consciousness and what we call the "self" has changed drastically through the generations. While we've discussed the ramifications of dualism, neuroscientist Antonio Damasio contemplates a modern approach to consciousness when writing, "There is indeed a self, but it is a process, not a thing, and the process is present at all times when we are presumed to be conscious."[14]

Fixed identities were abandoned with the discovery of neuroplasticity. People were empowered by the idea that we can change through a process of deprogramming and re-patterning. This not only changes the physical structure of our neural regions; it also shifts our attitude of what we call our "self." Every thought, feeling, and sensation begins and ends in our brain. And the language we use to describe it is often faulty. For example, we don't actually see with our eyes, hear with our ears, or taste with our tongues. Those organs send electrical impulses to our brains, which creates our perception of each sense. Our sense organs are transmitters; our brain translates.

So it is with every facet of existence. Siddhartha, the historical Buddha, was onto something when he claimed the self to be an illusion. Perhaps a better term is *construct*. In the ever-shifting nature of our ideas about our true nature, it is impossible to pinpoint an exact being. Words fail us. That is why in mindfulness meditation the first step is to recognize thoughts as thoughts, a more challenging prospect than it first appears. It is just a movement, but where it moves us, most often to the past or future, creates a sense of disembodiment. Understand how thoughts move and you learn to move them where you want them to go.

Think about it this way: your brain produces thoughts from the moment you wake up until you go to bed. Your idea of your self is inextricably bound up in these neuronal firings. Even while asleep your brain is thinking. Researchers have discovered that dreaming plays a pivotal role in memory consolidation.[15] Your brain consolidates your experiences, finding context based upon what you've already learned. This all happens without the *you* that you recognize as you doing anything—the illusion of the self. Even while awake we feel like our thoughts are "just happening" without conscious intervention. The neuroscientist Sam Harris discusses this phenomenon when writing, "It is not within our power to stop talking to ourselves, whatever the stakes. It's not even in our power to recognize each thought as it arises in consciousness without getting distracted every few seconds by one of them."[16]

Without meditation, Harris continues, it is impossible to remain aware of anything for more than a few moments at a time. This is what our brain does: it thinks, ceaselessly, relentlessly. It fluctuates. Our self is an attempt to recognize coherency in these fluctuations.

These fluctuations result in what we call consciousness. Neuroscientist Dan Levitin reminds us that consciousness is not a thing or even localizable in the brain. There is no "consciousness center." He writes, "It's simply the name we put to ideas and perceptions that enter the awareness of our central executive, a system of very limited capacity that can generally attend to a maximum of four or five things at a time."[17]

Richard Metzinger argues that the philosophical term *transparency* is necessary for understanding consciousness: we don't understand the mechanism transporting information to us. Just because we can't see it, though, does not mean the mechanisms are not understandable. It will just take a bit more time and research. Metzinger writes, "We do not see the window but only the bird flying by. We do not see neurons firing away in our brain but only what they represent for us."[18]

The true mystery of consciousness is how a small gelatinous organ that consumes 20 percent of our body's energy attempts to understand itself. Part of the reason we have so much time for thought is that the body's operating system is autonomic, taken care of below the level of our conscious understanding. Since the "construction process is largely invisible,"[19] we fill in the gaps of awareness with spirits, gods, and sundry ambitions, wonderful images created by our vast imagination. Yet even Patanjali recognized that our brains could easily be filled with false pretenses. Like Siddhartha, he knew that we suffer because we don't perceive reality correctly. Contemplating existence thousands of years before brain scans, he understood that humans believe their thoughts represent all of reality, and that we pay an emotional toll when realizing that's not the case. Instead of using our thoughts wisely, we become used by them. The gift of consciousness grows distraught by its own trappings. The self we construct imprisons us.

Patanjali also realized an escape from this prison exists. As meditation is the key, let's unlock the door.

THE PROGRAM: MEDITATION

Meditation #1: Minding Your Business

Like "consciousness," the term "mindfulness" has been widely defined. I like Sam Harris's definition: "It is simply a state of clear, nonjudgmental, and undistracted attention to the contents of consciousness, whether pleasant or unpleasant."[20] He writes that the word is derived from the Pali term *sati*, which means "clear awareness." Put simply, it is noticing what's going on inside of your head right now.

Earlier I mentioned that thoughts seem to just happen. Of course, there are many "places" they come from, just as they are influenced by your environment, your posture, what you ate today, and so forth. Mindfulness meditation is an opportunity to engage with the moment and witness your inner processes. The more proficient you become, the more you can control your reaction to your thoughts. You can practice mindfulness anywhere at any time: sitting, standing, walking, eyes open or closed. I find that sitting on a comfortable cushion—I use a pouf from a trip to Morocco—with my eyes closed offers me a wonderful opportunity to dive in. And like in the earlier workouts, I have a space in my apartment set aside for this. Find what works for you.

1. Sit comfortably on the ground or in a chair. Close your eyes and tune into your breathing for a few moments. Notice the quality and quantity of your breathing. Usually as the quantity decreases, the quality increases. Slow, measured breathing is the best way to still your mind and observe the present moment.

2. Think. Our brain produces thoughts constantly; don't try to stop the process. Simply observe what thoughts arise.

3. Observe the observed. One of my favorite sentiments from Buddhism: the observer observing the observed. That's Buddhist talk for metacognition. You're watching your own process. The trick here—the hard part—is to not become distracted by your thoughts. Don't create a narrative. If you

think about what you ate for breakfast, try not to contemplate dinner, as that's in the future. If an ex appears in your head, don't jump down that rabbit hole. Simply think to yourself, *oh, there's a thought. How interesting.* Then tap back into your breath and see what comes up next. Shoot for five minutes and soon ten will feel effortless. Don't overextend your visit, but don't allow yourself to break your meditation at the first distraction. They will happen. Use your breath as a tool to break through any fidgeting, boredom, or anxiety.

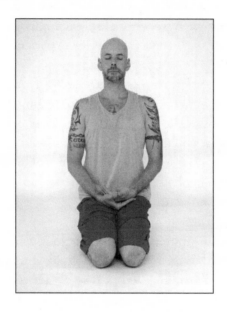

Meditation #2: Break on Through

This meditation asks you to imagine the pain of others in order to come to terms with your own capacity for empathy and healing. This is not an easy meditation, especially if you feel vulnerable. Yet I personally believe that's the *best* time to practice, given that a sense of hurt is prevalent. Meditation is not an escape but an entrance. Inspired by the Tibetan practice of *tonglen*, which means "taking and receiving," the most famous purveyor of this meditation is the Buddhist nun Pema Chödrön. This format is designed to strengthen your brain's resilience system. It is also the meditation I used when going through a divorce and cancer. In both situations it helped me manage the darkness I had entered and come through the other side stronger.

Hormesis is the phenomenon used to describe the act of creating tension to gain strength. This meditation works in a similar manner. You're momentarily injecting an emotional toxin to build resistance. The end game is not only helping yourself, but being more open with others. As Richard J. Davidson writes, "Part of an empathic response is feeling someone's pain. Indeed, recent research has shown that when we empathize, the brain activates many of the same networks as when we ourselves experience pain, physical or otherwise."[21]

Remember, you're merely introducing a small amount of toxin into your inner network of thoughts and feelings to emerge stronger. When you disassociate the *feeling* of psychic pain with the *content* that produces it, you come to terms with your inner world in startling new ways. By envisioning the pain of others you heal your own, developing a better relationship not only with yourself, but with those around you.

1. Find a comfortable seat. Closing your eyes, visualize someone who is suffering. It could be a child you saw on the news or a loved one dealing with a disease. Or it could be your own pain in the form of someone else's body. I've personally found better success imagining people I know; it is easier to relate to them. At the same time, if it's too close to home, invoking a random person might be a better option. If it is your own pain the figure can be shadowy or incomplete. What's important is that you recognize an entity in your mind's eye.
2. With every inhalation, picture yourself breathing in this person's pain, physical or existential. Envision that pain traveling through your nostrils, into your lungs, and radiating to all edges of your body.
3. As you exhale, imagine the pain leaving your body. Notice the sensation as your body is alleviated of suffering.

4. Repeat for at least twenty breaths, longer if you can sustain your focus. Over time the number of breaths won't matter, but in the beginning it's helpful to have a stable number to focus on. When complete, sit still for a few moments longer before opening your eyes again. Notice the shift in your feelings.

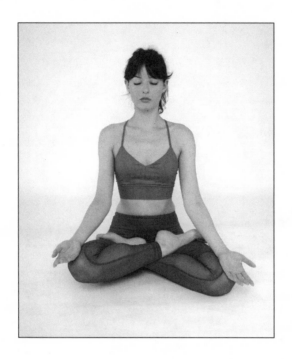

With time and patience this meditation weakens the connection between your amygdala, your fight-flight-freeze region, and prefrontal cortex, the center of rational thinking. A space appears between the time you have an emotion and your reaction. I like to think of the scene in *The Matrix* in which Neo dodges bullets in slow motion. With the creation of this distance between emotion and reaction, you're empowered to fill it with whatever you'd like. Choose wisely.

PART III
Mind

Chapter 9

The Art of Disruption

"If you believe you can change—if you make it a habit—the change becomes real. This is the real power of habit: the insight that your habits are what you choose them to be."

—Charles Duhigg, *The Power of Habit*

CHANGING AN INDUSTRY

When my doctor asked if I was driving, I knew the call was about to go downhill. The concern in her voice had already given away the test results. The tumor is indeed cancerous, she tells me. At this point I'm sitting on the floor in my living room, gut churning, shoulders seized. I do my best not to cry, a task I fail at when I call my father. The timeline is astounding: I feel the tumor Monday morning, and that afternoon I'm in my doctor's office; Tuesday morning, I'm at the radiologist, and by the afternoon I have a diagnosis. For all the complaints about the sluggish nature of the medical industry, cancer is one disease they take quite seriously.

While I knew that the chance of my being fine from testicular cancer was nearly guaranteed—against doctoral advice I searched online, though in my defense I stuck to PubMed—my life had been disrupted. Provided that I came through this unscathed—one surgery to remove the testicle and one round of chemotherapy did the trick—I would soon be a survivor. Over the next few months there was time off work due to surgical recovery and a month-long post-chemo focus on nutrition and immune system rebuilding. I feel fortunate that it was that manageable, this jab at mortality.

Disruption is usually something that happens to us: an accident, a disease, unemployment, heartbreak. Life is going along until a shift occurs. We can't control these events though we have a say in how we respond. Our emotions and mental state depend on our reaction to challenging circumstances. In the last chapter we looked at one discipline that helps reactivity. Now we're shifting gears.

In this section of the book we're focusing on disruptions we consciously choose. As an example, students often tell me they want strong abdominal muscles. As a concept, that's great. Putting in the work is usually the last thing they want to do, however. I see their faces during slow mountain climbers, plank variations, and boat pose flows. In fact, I know how my own face looks when I'm practicing these techniques. Here, however, we put our heads down and plow ahead.

Disruption has been an important word in the technology sector for decades. A primary goal of companies is to create a product or app that completely changes culture. One famous example is the iPhone. Telecommunications corporations laughed at Steve Jobs when he announced Apple was invading their territory. Yet he never intended to create a phone to compete with them. Instead, he invented a small computer that happens to make phone calls. An entire industry was disrupted.

More recently, disruption has been a fitness buzzword. The Movement Section is about disrupting movement patterns to introduce variety for optimal health. Now we move on to your mind. Of course, this is not an either/or scenario. We operate a whole-body system. In this section we'll investigate another side of fitness, namely what you're doing when not exercising. Inspired to create healthier and more diverse movement patterns, we'll look at creating better patterns for your home and work life by investigating nutrition, flow states, music, and attention. But first we need to understand what disruption entails and how that plays into the bigger scope of interacting with our environment. We begin with a trait every one of us practices every day: habits.

TURNING THE KEYSTONE

Charles Duhigg believes a three-step loop explains habits: cue-routine-reward. Environmental or emotional stimulation creates an automatic response; a habitual pattern commences; a reward is achieved.[1] The *New York Times* journalist notes that nearly half of what we believe to be conscious decision-making is really just a habit playing out.

I'll share an embarrassing story to highlight just how deeply ingrained habits are. Twice a week I teach yoga at the Beverly Hills Equinox. The underground parking deck is a bit of a nightmare given how many people attend the club. While parking rates are astronomical, members and employees get their ticket stamped; the first two hours are free. Since I often take a class before teaching (or sometimes teach back-to-back), I pay a discounted fee of one dollar for the extra hour.

One evening I arrive to find out the downstairs ticket machine is broken. I'm told that I just have to present the ticket on the way out and facility staff will open the gate upstairs. I take a class then teach mine. When I'm done I head to the machine where you slide your ticket in to pay. (The upstairs gate is usually automated.) An attendant reminds me that I just need to hand my ticket to the person upstairs as I'm leaving. I had admittedly forgotten, but here he is saving me the hassle. Even though he's telling me this, and even though I hear him and understand what he's saying, I slide my ticket in. And even though I know the most my fee has ever been is one dollar, I take the credit card out of my wallet and pay the $22 it would have cost if I was not affiliated with Equinox. He stands there staring at me. By the time I realize what I've done my card has been charged. It hits me all at once. The attendant tells me they might reimburse me upstairs, but at this point I'm too ashamed to even try. As someone whose life is all about pointing these things out,

I'm flabbergasted. I'm also out an additional twenty-one bucks. Yet I'm also human, prone to habitual patterns, like sliding a ticket into a machine. It was a humbling moment.

From an evolutionary perspective, habit formation is economical. Think about how we learn new skills. At first it takes quite a bit of effort. Once it becomes routine—riding a bike, driving to work, tying our shoelaces—we free up cognitive resources to focus on other tasks. This is a rather convenient function of neurobiology. But we also become stuck in ruts when the habits are unhealthy, or shake our head in disbelief when a pattern plays out even when we know better.

Neuroplasticity is our ability to change neural pathways and experience life differently. But the neurons that previously fired and wired together must be changed. Duhigg noticed that the only way to successfully change is by disrupting the second part of the loop: routine. Cues are often unavoidable; once we become accustomed to a reward, we're always going to want it. Our only recourse is to change our routines. That way, when we receive a cue and expect a reward, we can still achieve it.

This does not mean the reward will be exactly the same. The extreme end of pattern formation is addiction. Consider one of the most pervasive. The reward of alcohol is a certain feeling associated with the substance. It might be a physical high or an emotional escape. Regardless, alcohol disrupts the communication pathways in our brain, altering how we feel and think. It suppresses the amino acid glutamate, the most abundant neurotransmitter in the human nervous system, which affects memory and learning as well as serving as an important relay messenger for movement—hence, the loss of coordination. Alcohol also increases the effects of the neurotransmitter GABA, which reduces neuronal excitability and plays a role in muscle tone, further staggering your swagger.[2] Finally—this is key for the reward portion of the loop—alcohol floods your brain's reward center with dopamine.

While a few select people might crave a paunch and enjoy stumbling, most humans seek that dopamine fix, which is why cardiovascular exercise is a potent response to curbing alcohol addiction.

Running, cycling, and, if you're Don Draper, swimming are wonderful ways to change the routine. You still have a cue—you want to feel good—and the reward remains a dopamine rush. This is a simplistic view of addiction; the neurochemistry is much more insidious. But the basic premise is solid. Indeed, cardiovascular exercise and intense yoga disciplines like Kundalini have helped numerous addicts transform their lives.

Making such a switch does not have to be daunting. Forget addiction. Let's say you want to lose the growing visceral fat around your midsection. We'll talk nutrition in the next chapter, which is the most important factor in losing weight, but from a movement perspective one of the most efficient ways of shedding excess is running. Knowing this, you want in. You need a new routine. In this case, adding a cue might be beneficial. So you put your running shoes next to your bed instead of leaving them in your closet. Such a seemingly simple fix is highly effective. Removing the candy dish from the table in the office kitchen disrupts a cue that results in better (or less) snacking. Waking up to the sight of sneakers is a reminder you can't ignore. These "small wins," as Duhigg calls them, result in lasting progress. In fact, he writes that these "keystone habits" have a cascading effect. For example, people who start running tend to make better decisions in other aspects of their health, such as eating and sleeping better and gaining more control over their emotions. Sometimes it's just a matter of understanding where that keystone fits into the structure of your life.

Our brains always seek the easiest path. Unfortunately that's part of what habit formation is. We become accustomed to doing something a certain way, tricking ourselves into believing that's the most effective use of our time. Now, to counter this, we *are* quick learners. If someone points out an easier method we'll quickly change our tune. But then *that* becomes a habit, becoming just as ingrained.

This new habit, in many situations, seems to be the best thing for us. Until it's not. Look at the disruption capabilities of the driving app, Waze. You take the same route to work every day, unconsciously driving along the highway listening to your favorite podcast (mine is Revisionist History). Suddenly, you run into a wall of traffic you've never seen before. The cause is a bad accident, though you're miles away from understanding that. With a flick of a finger you're exposed to roads you've never imagined existed. Most people sit on the highway begrudgingly waiting it out. You don't have to. Like Duhigg writes in the opening quote to this chapter, you have to make a change in habit. Change damaging habits to healthier ones. What that entails is individual to each person, though I want to spend the rest of this chapter exploring a few everyday habits so ingrained and unconscious we don't even realize the potential damage we're doing.

TRIBAL ANIMALS

For years I taught a teacher-training module on neuroscience and yoga philosophy at Strala Yoga in New York City. During one session I mention a pet peeve: watching people ignore cashiers because they're too wrapped up in whatever's going on with their phone. Store clerks are treated like mere cogs in a machine, almost an inconvenience for the harried customer to escape from as quickly as possible to continue texting, reading, or chatting about, well, usually nothing. I reflected back to my years working in customer service, thankful I never had to deal with such disrespect from the people I served. I've often wondered how workers today feel. On occasion, when someone in front of me acts rudely, I ask. The cashier never expresses pleasure.

We break. Twenty minutes later, one of the women in the training asks if she can tell a story. During our break she went to a nut and candy shop on Broadway. While her phone is usually in her hand wherever she goes, she decided to leave it in the studio after what I had just expressed. With numerous choices in the store she asks the clerk for guidance. Before he responds he thanks her for taking the time out to talk to him. "I've been here all day, and you're the first person that hasn't been staring at their phone. I was beginning to feel like I'm not human."

In conversation and on social media we tend to focus on big-picture items, such as climate change, animal rights, politics, water conservation, and drug addiction. Rarely do we dive into minutiae. Let's step back for a moment and consider these questions:

- How often do you use Ziploc baggies?
- Do you realize that plant agriculture kills more animals and destroys more habitats than many animal facilities?
- What is the name of your district's representative?
- Do you leave the faucet or shower running while you shave?
- How much sugar do you consume in a day?

When thinking of climate change, we'll post photos of ice caps melting thanks to carbon emissions. How could *my* plastic bag affect the planet? As for animals, most destroyed by combines and other large-scale machines are insects and small mammals, not the larger, more evolved creatures that I love. Do they really count?

Wait, my district has a representative?

Of course many of us do realize these details, such as our voice in local government. Then again, given the number of men letting the faucet run while shaving at the gym you'd think California wasn't experiencing the worst drought in state history—thousands of years of history, in fact. Part of the problem involves believing problems are created by "other" people out there. Yet we all play a role in society. Whether we realize it or not, by being a member of a collective we've signed an unspoken contract for conduct and practices. This is why numerous Americans become so frustrated by how few taxes corporations pay. Our nation's infrastructure, health care, and security depend on our contribution. When someone bucks the system while we're still paying it's hard not to feel anger and resentment.

There are many unspoken contracts we share that are rarely discussed. They usually fall under the category of ethics, a discipline most leave behind once the section on Aristotle in school has been covered. Morality, however, is what culture hinges upon—religions and governments alike define ethical boundaries; public perception of fairness depends on these rules. This is not only social; it's biological. Behavior is passed along in the genetic code, not what we think or how we feel (though thoughts and emotions do influence behavior).[3] Since the functioning of society depends on interaction, when the various parts—the people—act in unhealthy ways, the structure crumbles. Seemingly innocuous events like disregarding a teller or consuming a hundred grams of sugar every day add up. An ignored person begins ignoring (or lashing out) at others; health care rates skyrocket as more citizens are diagnosed with type 2 diabetes. As basic as this sounds, being nice and paying attention to others goes a long way, often undetectably. Doing unto others—that whole bit.

A society is like a body. While dynamical systems theory is usually applied to planetary orbits and electronic circuits, in biomechanics it serves as a framework for understanding the dependent connections of our regulatory systems: how breathing influences thinking, for example, or how blood circulation affects our nervous system. When one part of one system begins to fail, the effects are system-wide. Parkinson's disease begins with bodily shaking and rigidity but soon affects all motor behavior, as well as speaking and thinking. Depression and anxiety are common at the onset, which further instigate the disease's problems. Anyone who has had a family member with Alzheimer's understands this cascading demise as well.

Culturally we immediately recognize who the outliers are, such as terrorists and mass murderers. Most people do not act in such a manner. We aim to lead fulfilling, meaningful lives. But if the scope of our awareness is pointed only at our own ambitions and goals influenced by the whims of our temperament, the larger picture is fragmented into many tiny pieces. Tribes with under a hundred and fifty members would never act in such a manner; their existence depended upon cooperation. Hierarchies were generally shunned, and if any alpha grew too drunk on power he was quickly knocked down to size (or disposed of for the good of the group).

Things are not so simple in cities with millions of citizens. Even though talk of tribes and evolutionary biology sounds whimsical, we live with challenging contradictions as we're still operating with the same tribal impulses. The problem is the structure of our lifestyles is vastly different. I could feasibly live an entire year without leaving my apartment. I'd have to give up teaching public classes, but since a large portion of my income is made online through writing and editing, and since all my groceries could be delivered to my front door, I could easily shack up and become a hermit. This is truly unprecedented in human history. No one in their right mind would want to live such an existence. Tribal implies social; it's the genetic code we come pre-wired with. Acting as though we're individual islands is where the disparity resides. This habit of self-enclosure is what we need to disrupt if we want to grow personally and culturally.

This is no easy task. You most likely purchased this book because you want to have more energy, be more flexible, or lose weight. These are all valuable goals that also have cascading effects. Look someone in the eye, and try to tell him or her to get off his or her phone. The blowback can inspire vitriol. People don't like being told what to do. But as I said early on in this book, we have to put *everything* on the table. The health of society is interdependently entwined with personal health. In the end, people aren't going to remember you for how many pull-ups you can do or whether or not you can press into a handstand. The value of your character *will* be remembered. That might involve disrupting more important habits than any physical program can offer.

One of the most challenging disruptions humans face in the modern era is in their food choices. Never before has so much food been available at one time. This has resulted in a variety of mismatch diseases and consumer confusion. It is also a deeply personal topic, as what we put into our bodies becomes part of us. I've never received so much resistance and ideological pontification as with food, and for good reason: you are what you eat (or, as Michael Pollan writes, you are what you eat eats; or, as our pre-cooking ancestors would have said, you are what you'd rather not eat[4]). Societies are structured on diet; cultures lean heavily on culinary traditions for sustenance and identity; the chemistry of nutrition informs our deepest sense of self. Tell someone they eat too much or that they eat poorly? Receive a tongue lashing of divine fury. Question a vegan's ethics? How dare you. Suggest foie gras and veal devotees repent on ethical grounds? Blasphemous hippie.

As we're discussing health, there is no more important factor than what we put into our bodies. What's on your table influences your brain and body more than anything else. While an encyclopedia would be needed to address such a vast topic, we'll briefly touch upon important research on disrupting eating habits next.

Chapter 10

What Goes In ...

"Is there any more futile, soul-irradiating experience than standing before the little window on a microwave oven watching the carousel slowly revolve your frozen block of dinner?"

—Michael Pollan, *Cooked*

PATTERNS OF SUBSISTENCE

We started our movement journey as unicellular beings. Energy production—that's what food is at the cellular level—begins here. But we won't revisit the evolutionary biology lesson. Instead, let's start with a romanticized narrative that rewinds us ten thousand years to the Fertile Crescent, the seat of agriculture and cradle of civilization. This is where humans domesticated themselves in a vast stretch of the Middle East. The notion of one region as the birthplace of farming fits this mindset. The problem is that crop and animal domestication occurred spontaneously around the planet. There were no satellite farmers proselytizing from the Levant. Still, this particular cradle is where wheat was domesticated. It has been an essential component of the human diet ever since.

When did humans truly become modern? British biologist Colin Tudge pushes the ten-thousand-year theory back thirty thousand more to proto-farmers manipulating their environment to collect and store food. Archaeology professor Steven Mithen dates it back 1.8 million years, historian Yuval Noah Harari 2.5 million—our ancestors were more in tune with the natural world than any modern could imagine. Early humans were certain to have used plants to their advantage, just as they'd been doing with animal migrations. Tudge also disdains the notion of invention, writing, "People did not invent agriculture and shout for joy; they drifted or were forced into it, protesting all the way."[1]

Why would hunter-gatherers resist domestication? Habit played a role. If you're accustomed to foraging, hunting, gathering, and otherwise being active, your ethos includes diversity by default. Tending to the monotony of crop cycles must have seemed demeaning. Tudge's proclaimed opposition hints at more than overcoming patterns. Climate change is one convincing argument, although humans long endured atmospheric shifts over the eons without settling down. Mithen believes the timing of this particular climate disruption coupled with advanced toolmaking techniques provides a missing link. As technological advancements aided harvesting and gathering, Natufian culture in the Levant became what is recognized as the first semi-sedentary society, preparing upcoming generations for lifetimes of backbreaking labor with little reward and no glory.

Then there's the perspective of movement, which doesn't necessarily contradict these ideas; there is rarely only one cause for anything. In the first section of this book I argued that movement is our evolutionary birthright, right down to our thinking. To move anything we need fuel. It's hard to imagine an entire people voluntarily deciding to stop roaming. It had been part of their DNA for two million-plus years. Why farming, then? As Tudge and others claim, a number of modern health problems began with widespread agriculture. Journalist Sebastian Junger writes, "Genetic adaptations take 25,000 years to appear in humans, so the enormous changes that came with agriculture in the last 10,000 years have hardly begun to affect the gene pool."[2] Yet affect us they have.

Did farming make life easier? Hardly. Besides having a major impact on economics—income disparity arose when an elite stored surplus crops, using food as bargaining chips—the life of a farmer, then and now, has never been without challenges. New infrastructure problems arose as humans settled into large villages and shared the duties required of farming: sanitation, depletion of resources, and social tension. Harvard paleoanthropologist Daniel Lieberman cites over one hundred mismatch diseases that came into existence when we transitioned to agriculture, including acid reflux, anxiety, osteoporosis, depression, cavities, and lower back pain.[3] Records show that early farmers suffered substantially poorer nutrition, experienced more disease and infections, and saw a reduction in life span compared to their hunting-gathering peers.[4] Add to this toxic mix a surge in war. If you want to defeat an enemy, cutting off (or stealing) their food supply is the quickest path to victory. Humans were violent animals before agriculture, but like technology exploiting our penchant for inattention today, crops exploited entire societies in ways previously unimaginable.

One key factor in nutrition, just like in movement, is variety. Eating an array of foods is essential. By the very nature of their lifestyle, hunter-gatherers munched on an assorted range of nutrients. (The Kalahari Desert's !Kung population, for example, eats 365 species of animals and plants.[5]) Monocropping would never have occurred to them. Sure, there were lean times, but crop failures, floods, and droughts ravaged cities and brought death on a large scale. One of the sad facts about Ireland's potato famine in the middle of the nineteenth century, responsible for the death of nearly two million citizens, was the abundance of readily available wild grasses and vegetables. They just didn't know where to look. Imagine New York suddenly cut off from food imports or a devastating earthquake knocking out water pipelines streaming into Los Angeles. How would we survive today?

With every form of nutrition available to us year-round, habits still predominate. To compensate for poor diets we turn to the gym, expecting the growing band of visceral fat around our middle to disappear on the treadmill. Or we limit caloric intake without recognizing nutrients matter more than number of calories. While essential vitamins and micronutrients, such as vitamins B12, A, E, and D, cholesterol, magnesium, and iron, are readily available in the supermarket produce section, we'd rather take a multi-vitamin. I'm not against multi-vitamins per se, but the efficacy of dousing yourself without knowing exactly what your body lacks is a questionable way to achieve health.

There has never been a time in history that markets offered so much for so little. For most of the world's population, starvation is not a concern. We've swung the pendulum in the other direction. America, along with many other nations, struggles with obesity. While there is evidence that this problem has leveled off thanks to public awareness initiatives and a concerted focus on organic agriculture and grass-fed protein, the social and economic impact remains steep. In 2008 the Center for Disease Control put an annual price tag of obesity at $147 billion.[6] This includes the burden on our health care system, absenteeism from work due to health issues related to obesity, and even the extra gasoline required to haul larger bodies around.

Governmental agencies have gotten a lot of information wrong in the past. This is to be expected. As science and technology develops, researchers investigate new territories and undue old assumptions. As obesity levels skyrocket, an insidious mixture of economics, social anxiety regarding thinner bodies, corporate interests, public skepticism, and dietary misinformation assault the American imagination. It's taken a half-century to rewrite the story of nutritive health. Yet all it really took was rewinding the clock ten millennia.

BACK TO THE FUTURE

While innumerable events have had planetary consequences, the reverberations of World War II arguably rank amongst consequences that are still being felt the strongest. This battle forced each nation to self-reflect. Are we tribal or global? Is the extermination of religious and ethnic groups morally sound? Should we allow scientists to tinker with the genetic code? That last question is still being asked (and debated) thanks to an increasing field of knowledge.

While many horrors were unearthed during that era— concentration camps; biological experiments that informed dystopian science fiction; the destructive power of atomic energy—a decisive march toward multiculturalism resulted. In addition to the uniting of previously disparate religious and ethnic groups, another effect is that women firmly embedded themselves in the American workforce. Soldiers returning home expecting their wives to return to the kitchen received a rude awakening.

Enter capitalism. The frozen food industry and fast food businesses were there for the family. Clever advertising campaigns promised more free time by unshackling both men and women (though predominantly women) from the slave labor of kitchen duty. Two hours for dinner? Try twenty minutes. Remove from freezer, pop into oven, get back to television. Or have him pick it up on the way home from work. You deserve it.

Freezing food was not new. A thousand years ago the Chinese preserved edibles in ice cellars. Electricity eventually discarded the need for underground storage. An ingenious Canadian engineer named Clarence Birdseye solved the problem of food transportation between world wars. As World War II commenced, Americans were buying eight hundred million pounds of frozen food every year.[7] Emerging corporations took a cue from airlines by packaging ready-made dinners in aluminum trays. Swanson sold ten million TV dinners when launching in 1954.

Humans are natural problem solvers. Imagine a problem and someone will find the solution. Envisioning our way out of tight places is a feature of our neural networks. One reason humans have been so successful during our evolutionary course is our imagination. Ingenuity is a critical quality in an uncertain world. Like mass production, food preservation gave us a leg up. Certain chemical reactions, like those in fermented foods, have proven exceptional for our gut's microbiome, the trillions of microbes inhabiting our digestive system. One of the most exciting areas of research today is the enteric nervous system, your stomach's direct line to your brain. Some specialists believe this system is even more impactful on our health than the central nervous system. Just as we are the stuff of stars at a cellular level, the food we consume becomes us.

This is a problem when the nutrients we ingest no longer nourish, as has been the case with most processed foods. Fermented foods naturally have a long shelf life. Chemicals that extended the life of perishable foods alter our microbiome in disastrous ways. Now two major problems are making us sick and overweight. First, humans are creatures of habit. Available food options might be plentiful, but many people stick to a limited range of items. More problematic is the nutritional make-up of those limited foods. We know that sugar is as addictive as cocaine and nicotine.[8] Clever marketers have engineered a process to sidestep this dilemma. These food producers know another route to get sugar into our body under the guise of dozens if not hundreds of names. Yet they mostly return to one: carbohydrates.

IT'S NOT THAT COMPLEX

Mismatch diseases are chronic ailments that have resulted thanks to what we call civilization. Evolution does not necessarily make a species better. Adaptability is the secret ingredient of biology; humans have simply not adapted well to many so-called advances. Every change in the genetic code requires mutation, but a mutation is not the cause of a disease. As physician and author Siddhartha Mukherjee writes, "The definition of disease rests, rather, on the specific disabilities caused by an *incongruity* between an individual's genetic endowment and his or her current environment—between a mutation, the circumstances of a person's existence, and his or her goals for survival or success. It is not mutation that ultimately causes disease, but mismatch."[9]

One telling mismatch involves something many of us extracted during youth. While it appears evolution did us a disservice with "extra" teeth, molars were once critical for chewing. There are innumerable benefits to cooking food, including an increased energy load and an external means of breaking down nutrients to ease the digestive process. This softness allows us to chew less. In many ways this is important to the functioning of society. Primates spend up to six hours a day laboriously chomping tubers, stems, roots, and leaves. For us, five minutes on a stovetop then another five in the bowl lets us get on with our day. Since we no longer stress our faces the way our ancestors did, our jaws have adapted, which is why these teeth are unnecessary and even painful.

Many of us don't masticate enough to begin with. Chewing plays many important roles in digestion, including breaking down complex carbohydrates into simple ones. Where cooking meets agriculture turns out to be the intersection of our greatest maladies. The modern diet is filled with complex carbs in the forms of corn, wheat, potatoes, rice, and other grains. Fruits and vegetables also contain complex carbs, though in much smaller amounts. We often associate fruit with sugar intake, outside of added sugars, of course. This lack of foresight allows the insidiousness of industrial farming and monocropping to rear their ugly heads.

Sugars are simple carbohydrates. Chewing is the catalyst for the transformation of denser, complex carbs. Bite by bite you're breaking down these molecules. With over 260 different names for that sweet mixture of fructose and glucose, humans consume sugar at mind-boggling rates; currently the average American consumes 152 pounds of it every year.[10] Add to that 146 pounds of flour—complex turns simple—and we're witnessing a mismatch of calamitous proportions. Among the numerous ailments that can be directly traced to overconsumption of sugar, type 2 diabetes, obesity, and heart disease top the list. Add in strokes, high blood pressure, and even some forms of cancer. Throw in a number of tooth diseases for good measure.

Knowing the dangers of sugar has not curbed our appetite for it. Consider the public vitriol against initiatives like Michael Bloomberg's failed attempt to limit the serving sizes of sugary beverages—which result in the death of 184,000 people each year[11]—in which New York City residents rallied against the supposed infringement of their freedom. We certainly have an odd definition of freedom if by that word we mean allowing damaging addictions to overrule common sense and public health. Regardless, there are many books that rail against the dangers of sugar, as well as a growing body of research as to how carbohydrates break down into sugar inside your body. For the rest of this chapter I'd like to argue for a solution.

TIME TO DETOX

It is impossible to study the traditions of India without considering vegetarianism. Despite the idealistic notion of being early ethicists—there is evidence that the ban on eating animals was in part sanctioned by an elite class installing dietary restrictions, i.e., you get the vegetables, we get the meat—it is undeniable that Indians were early in the veg-only camp. Influenced by this I gave up beef at eighteen, pork at nineteen, and all the rest at twenty-one, save seafood, which remained a part of my diet until I was thirty. Then, for moral and health reasons, I committed to full vegetarianism for a decade, including two years of veganism.

I'm not going to touch the moral side of this argument, as it is beyond the scope of this book. From a health perspective, I was misguided. I don't attribute this solely to meat consumption, though I am no longer vegetarian. Rather, I was a carb junkie. Most of my calories came from vegetables and grains, in the form of quinoa, millet, rice, and so much bread.

I consider myself a healthy person. I teach and practice fitness and yoga six days a week. Despite constant and varied movement, I suffered many lingering issues. I graduated college around 175 pounds in 1997; by age forty I was 185 pounds. At a height of six-three, this is not a heavy load to carry, though I did notice, year by year, a slight increase in the midsection of the body. No matter how much cardio or lifting I did, it would not budge. Like many other men I accepted it as an inevitability of aging.

There *are* certainly inevitabilities in life, but a required "pound a year" of visceral fat is not one of them. In January 2016 I gave up grains and integrated high-quality protein back into my life. I also focused on fats. The results were stunning. Within three weeks I was back down to 175. The puffiness in my body relented. Chronic gastritis, which I had been dealing with for two decades, was reduced by 90 percent. Lingering inflammation from surgeries in my right shoulder and left knee, as well as new trouble spots in my elbows, mostly disappeared. I slept better. Chronic canker sores were gone. And, perhaps most surprisingly, I stopped having anxiety attacks. Since age sixteen I've suffered hundreds of attacks, including two ending in a hospital visit and one that caused me to black out, walk into a wall, and wake up on some poor woman's lap in an East Village restaurant. In my early thirties I spent half a year on Xanax; yoga and meditation helped me off meds. It was not until I changed my diet that my anxiety dissipated. To be clear, I still have moments of anxiety, but since quitting the carb-heavy diet, none have resulted in an attack. If you've suffered one, you know the difference.

This evidence is entirely anecdotal and should be treated as such. But I did not make a personal decision like the above without research. By adopting a fat-heavy, moderate-carb diet, I feel like I've acquired a new body. I'm not alone in this journey. This combination has resulted in incredible results for many people concerned about their well-being.

Language plays a fundamental role in our confusion. When one word takes on multiple meanings, we tend to confuse the two. Fat is one such word. Of course, one is a less kosher version of obesity. But fat is so much more. It is one of three macronutrients necessary for survival, alongside carbohydrates and protein. At nine calories per gram, fat is much more efficient for energy than protein or carbs, each of which has four.

For decades it has been believed that eating fat makes you fat, so avoid it at all costs. Yet fat is how we became humans to begin with. Along with the social currency afforded by banding together in tribal communities, an ability to stockpile fat is how our forebears "evolved big brains and slow-growing bodies."[12] Dietary fat was, for most of our history, secured whenever possible. As our stockpiles grew more abundant, our psychology flipped. Despite decades of avoiding fat, including the production of a godless amount of low-fat food products, we've only gotten fatter. Something is wrong.

In what is known as the "American paradox," researchers have long been miffed by how the French consume so much butter and fat yet remain slender. They also experience relatively low levels of heart disease—the main culprit implicated in the anti-fat crusade. Americans, by contrast, have spent over a half-century removing fat from our diets only to watch waistlines grow, mismatch diseases skyrocket, and death rates soar. Tragically, this misinformation originated with the work of one stubborn man.

Ancel Keys created the K-rations diet, helpful to soldiers during World War II, as well as the Mediterranean diet. He offered critical evidence regarding nutrition and fasting. At times his ego was bigger than his discernment, however. His crusade against fat began with one study involving thirty men from Crete. Keys surveyed their previous day's diet. He then investigated data from other countries in which more saturated fat was being consumed. Since the men from Crete suffered fewer heart attacks, Keys believed this limited information inferred causation.

Keys gathered data from six countries that backed up his belief that fats are bad. The problem is he left out details from sixteen nations that contradicted this evidence. Soon after, he launched his famous Seven Countries Study, again cherry-picking countries that fit his narrative. He has also been criticized for not including carbohydrate or sugar levels when investigating the amount of fat being consumed. This remains a problem today. For example, we think of hamburgers as terrible when the actual horror involves the quality (and quantity) of bread, amount of sugar in the condiments, and whether the cow was fed grass or grain. Nutrition is a complex relationship of numerous factors. Zeroing in on one without considering others is irresponsible.

These are external factors before the meal enters our body. From there, food becomes "information that radically influences our genes, hormones, immune system, brain chemistry, and even gut flora with every single bite."[13] Overanalyzing each bite is itself a disease known as orthorexia. I'm not counseling it. But consider this: bread, the staple food of the world since the advent of agriculture, requires four ingredients: flour, salt, water, and time. In an attempt to discard that last element, we—most likely, the bakery—add dozens of ingredients to bake bread as quickly as possible. All processed foods share a similar folklore. Get out of the kitchen and into, well, wherever isn't the kitchen. What we save in the moment we pay for later on.

Thus people go to insane lengths to lose weight instead of devoting more time to handling their food. While the pathway to digestion begins with teeth and saliva, catabolism explains the route inside. A set of metabolic processes that breaks down and oxidizes food molecules, this is how the chain of energy production begins. Sadly, the more we pack in, the more we affect how that chain functions. This is common when people lose weight. For example, Danny Cahill, a former contestant in the popular show "The Biggest Loser," is known as the "biggest loser ever" for dropping 239 pounds and winning the show. He describes how it happened: "Wake up at 5 a.m. and run on a treadmill for 45 minutes. Have breakfast—typically one egg and two egg whites, half a grapefruit, and a piece of sprouted grain toast. Run on the treadmill for another 45 minutes. Rest for 40 minutes; bike ride nine miles to a gym. Work out for two and a half hours. Shower, ride home, eat lunch— typically a grilled skinless chicken breast, a cup of broccoli, and ten spears of asparagus. Rest for an hour. Drive to the gym for another round of exercise."[14]

Like many big losers, Cahill gained much of the weight back. The above regimen is unsustainable—exercise has been shown to help little with weight loss[15], and over-exercising comes with its own problems. (Notice how he rests for an hour, but says nothing about regenerative practices, which also help weight loss.) On top of that his diet reflects the perfect pyramid of carb and sugar dependence (toast, grapefruit) and fat avoidance (egg whites, skinless chicken breast) that has been proffered as healthy.

In the publishing industry, the target audience for self-help books is people who have previously purchased self-help books. The same holds true for diet books, which indicates that people who go on a diet rarely stay on it, always searching for something else that works. What matters is that you *change* your diet, not that you diet. Like the word "fat," "diet" has two meanings, one dangerous to our psychology and emotional health. Counting calories does not help. Eating whole, unprocessed foods high in fat and low in carbs does.

In an over-processed, undernourished world, it really is simple: sugar is killing us. While the term "toxic" is overused and misunderstood—natural food companies liberally plaster the word on nearly any product—glucose truly deserves this word. Partner-in-crime to fructose, these two comprise the simple carbohydrates that get broken down on the journey to your throat. For the most part what we term sugar is half glucose, half fructose. Exact percentages vary; high-fructose corn syrup is 55 percent fructose, for example.

Glucose shoots straight into your bloodstream while its partner requires enzymes to transform it into glucose. From there it also enters your veins. How can this major fuel source be poisonous? Humans have eaten sugars forever. Details, details: even fruit does not hijack your bloodstream the way processed foodstuffs do. (We've also selected sweeter fruits for reproduction and left the more fibrous, denser strains behind.) When glucose slides into your circulatory system, your pancreas secretes insulin to remove it from your bloodstream. Insulin is your body's security guard against toxicity. What happens at a concert when a crowd floods against the barrier? Security is overwhelmed. Bodies get crushed. The masses overthrow the government—or, in physiological parlance, type 2 diabetes. That blood sugar rush you enjoy after a pint of ice cream is your pancreas working triple time trying to rid your body of ice cream.

Not that this is *all* bad, mind you. Our bodies are incredibly adaptable. Upon ingestion, glucose is first shuttled off to your muscles and organs in the form of glycogen, which *is* fuel for movement (or thought, as our brains are tremendous energy suckers). This process only goes on for a few ounces of sugar. Then comes system overload. Your body converts excess glucose into fat, the bad word, predominantly stored around your belly, thighs, and butt. What constitutes too much? After years of political wrangling from the sugar lobby, the World Health Organization declared twenty-five grams of added sugar per day as the upper limit, meaning besides the naturally occurring sugars in fruits and veggies. This is less than the amount of sugar in a bottle of soda or an organic fresh-pressed juice. Sorry, juice junkies, one "detoxifying" green juice toxifies plenty (if your juicerista is liberal with bananas, apples, and pineapple). Considering one bottle of Naked's Green Machine contains a whopping fifty-three grams of sugar, you have to sip it for over two days to not breach the border. Even BluePrint fans who enjoy spending eleven dollars a bottle will be disappointed to learn that at twenty-two grams per Grass Monkey, you've pretty much hit your limit. Remember, this is total amount per day. You then have to figure in whatever else you're consuming.

Yes, glycogen fuels muscles and organs. While a little sugar goes a long way, fat goes longer. In fact, fat turns out to be a better source of energy production than glycogen. Humans have long consumed sugars and carbs as part of a balanced diet. The keys are variety and method of delivery. Fruit, for example, contains fiber, a substance our digestive system craves. Juicing strips insoluble fibers out, one of the main benefits of eating fruit. This is not to single out juice to give a free pass to other forms of sweetness. All metabolic syndromes are rooted in an overconsumption of sugars regardless of how they got inside. The trend of assigning certain sugars "organic" or "natural" is missing the point. Your mind might be comforted by organic sugarcane, but your body is going to treat it like cola.

There are actual devils and perceived ones. Carbs and sugars are mismatches; dietary fat is not. There is another word that has received much bad press over the decades. Keys's archenemy is cholesterol, the foundation of the multi-billion-dollar statins industry. Again he goes for simplicity: fats raise cholesterol levels; cholesterol leads to atherosclerosis, plaque build-up in your arteries; atherosclerosis leads to heart attacks and strokes and could kill you. So, bad cholesterol! And by implication, bad fats! It's unfortunate that the science is not that simple.

We know there are a number of fatty acids, which are chains of carbon, oxygen, and hydrogen atoms. Each acid is defined by how many carbon atoms live in each chain, as well the number of double bonds within each molecule. Fats with lots of double bonds are polyunsaturated. Fats with none are saturated. There are four types of fatty acids: saturated, monosaturated, polyunsaturated, and trans. Common wisdom has long promoted unsaturated fats, found in nuts, olive oil, and avocadoes, as heart-healthy, while the saturated fats found in meat have been demonized. Trans fat was invented by French chemist Paul Sabatier just over a century ago, but it was the German chemist Wilhelm Normann who first hydrogenated oils. This led to the creation of the first trans fat product: Crisco. As this fat is not found outside of the laboratory, it should be avoided completely. Nevertheless, the margarine movement was created to boost sales, not to promote good science. Beyond obesity, one 2011 study found a link between trans fats and depression.[16] The proper amount of trans fat to incorporate into your diet is none.

The real target of Keys and others has been saturated fats. This is odd, given that they are necessary for your nervous system to work, suppress inflammation, contain a range of essential vitamins, are required for the production of testosterone and estrogen, strengthen your immune system, and help you breathe better. Even more surprisingly, dietary saturated fats play *no role* in raising blood saturated fats.[17] Those levels are dictated by, you guessed it, carbs and sugars (as well as excess protein).

The conundrum of nutrition becomes even more confusing due to popular misunderstanding of low-density lipoproteins (LDL) and high-density lipoproteins (HDL), "bad" and "good" forms of cholesterol. While we assume that high LDL leads to heart and weight problems, a better marker is actually low HDL, which is the result of a low-fat, high-carbohydrate diet.[18] People with high dietary cholesterol do not necessarily experience heart attacks. What really matters is particle size. Small, dense LDL particles clog your arteries; light, airy HDL particles pass through without problem. Envision the difference between a golf ball and a beach ball, and ask yourself which one would hurt more if you were pegged with it.

Type of fat is more relevant than the amount of it. Yes, fat can be bad. Sadly, many studies do not take carb or sugar intake into consideration when denouncing those dastardly fats. Our ancestors ate a balanced blend of fat, carbs, and protein. Their lifestyles and technologies didn't allow for the hoarding of a single food source. The dawn of agriculture began a downward spiral in mono-cropping (and mono-eating), eventually facilitated by refrigeration and storage techniques coupled with nutrition science turning into nutritional engineering. A longtime quest to cook less and lounge more has resulted in deadly mismatch diseases. The good news is we can overturn this cycle of gradual decay by spending more time in the kitchen, handling the ingredients that go into the meals that become our bodies. This can become a communal affair by spending time with family and friends. There's something rewarding about lugging my overfilled bag home from the farmer's market. Participating in alchemical transformations to bring food to my plate is informative, primal, and healthy. Massaging greens for salad and kimchi, thinly slicing layers of onions, garlic, and peppers for soffritto, and slicing into a hearty striped bass are all means by which I connect to my bodily nourishment—not to mention brain nourishment, as that organ loves to be powered by fats. Knowing what spices and oils go into my food, as well as having a relationship with the farms from which I purchase my produce and meats, helps me stay on top of my health.

PRACTICE OF PATIENCE

There is no easy solution to the question of nutrition, but one thing is certain: patience is everything. Sadly, that's something we seem to be in shorter supply of than ever before.

America is obsessed with cooking shows despite the fact that we spend less time now preparing food than ever before—on average, we currently spend twenty-seven minutes a day.[19] We'd rather have cooks cook for us than cook for ourselves; we'll outsource meals to corporations and services whose bottom line has nothing to do with health. Ignorant of the oils and additives going into each meal—or, worse, failing to read the ingredient list to question why a loaf of bread requires thirty ingredients—nutrients we believe healthy are saturated with unsuspecting sugars and trans fats. Instead of changing our diet we default to our doctors, ingesting a cocktail of chemicals that mask but do not solve our internal dilemma, and in many cases create more chaos in regions we'll never see but that we feel every single day.

Then you have nutrition trends. We've mentioned the role of fats and cholesterol, but perhaps no greater perceived demon exists than gluten. And again, the problem might just be patience. In that suspect loaf of bread our cultural problem comes into view. By far the hardest subtraction from my diet is bread, a lifelong comfort food. Research shows that we prefer the foods we grew up eating,[20] and for me that's a loaf (along with eggs, though those fatty yolks are gold).

Many have eschewed bread for a gluten-free trend due to celiac disease. I suspect that a lot of this, like any other food trend, is hype. True, too many grains are not healthy; some people really have celiac disease and need to avoid bread. But what has caused this rampant increase in food allergies? Is it the quality of American wheat, which changed when former Secretary of Agriculture and corporate farming advocate Earl Butz encouraged farmers to plant "fencerow to fencerow" in the seventies? Possibly. But a more reasonable response might just be our impatience.

You know the frustrations of breadmaking if you've ever carefully kneaded and caressed dough for hours only to heave a dry loaf from the oven. Likewise, if you've ever spent a day massaging, proofing, and gazing at the wonders of fermentation and are rewarded with a springy, airy sourdough for dinner, you understand the absolute joy of the *boulanger*. Breadmaking is a meditation, a testament of patience, will, and fortitude. The dough does not lie. The mysterious alchemy of food comes to life in the oven. With so many factors beyond control, it's a wonder our ancestors figured out how to bake in the first place.

Yes, they probably had more time on their hands. Here again we trade time for health. As Michael Pollan writes, "Some researchers attribute the increase in gluten intolerance and celiac disease to the fact that modern breads no longer receive a lengthy fermentation."[21] Just as chewing breaks down food in our mouths and cooking breaks down chemicals into palatable nutrition, fermenting bread (among other foods) eases the digestive process. Sourdough fermentation destroys peptides responsible for celiac disease, while acids slow the absorption of sugars in your body, reducing the insulin spike carbohydrates cause. The mystery of bread is credited to airborne bacteria pervading our atmosphere—flour plus water and time harnesses these lively fellows. By contrast, baker's yeast comes only in one variety: *Saccharomyces cerevisiae*, selected for its ability to dependably make bread rise. Every manufactured bread relies on this singular strain. Bread, the closest food to divinity imaginable, the most produced and eaten substance around the planet for millennia, is having its way with us because we refuse to listen to what it needs.

Patience is everything. Your nervous system is not designed for constant input. Like movement, like media, you have to know what you're consuming. Nutrition affects not only our microbiome but our entire being. Discerning between marketing and health is hard when terms like "all natural" and "free range" are practically meaningless. We might not want to spend a lot of time thinking about food, but what we're replacing that time with—television, smart phones, binge-watching—is simply not worth the cost. Creating a connection with what you put in your body, a real hands-on means of touching, feeling, and sensing the plants and animals that you consume, is an essential part of reorienting your nervous system to create an optimal lifestyle. This is important, as your nervous system simply does not want to be on constant alert.

Chapter 11

Entering the Flow

"The best moments in our lives are not the passive, receptive, relaxing times . . . The best moments usually occur if a person's body or mind is stretched to its limits in a voluntary effort to accomplish something difficult and worthwhile."

—Mihaly Csíkszentmihályi, *Flow: The Psychology of Optimal Experience*

LEARNING TO FLY

On June 25, 2004, I stepped onto a small airplane. There were no seats; only a dozen of us boarded. We slid toward the front of the plane, holding onto a handrail. Slowly the plane climbed an early summer sky. Cloudy the entire day, around two the sky broke open, bright beams of sun filtering to a planet on which I was celebrating my twenty-ninth birthday—a planet I was climbing away from. A thousand feet. Two thousand. Five. Ten.

The coordinator tells us to prepare. A man slides behind me, snapping two buckles around my shoulders, two at my hips. I'm not usually this intimate with strangers. Then again I don't jump from the sky every day. Nearing thirteen thousand feet, we shuffle toward the door. The cold wind is assaulting. Thirteen-five. Let's go, he says.

There's no thinking. You can't contemplate what you're about to do, especially if you've never done it before. There's no frame of reference, nothing to guess or grab at. We leap. I assume a position similar to bow pose, a yogic backbend performed on the stomach. After a few spins we're righted, I think. I don't know. There's no way to explain freefalling. The human body was not designed to handle such circumstances. I'm watching the barometer strapped to my wrist for the moment we hit five thousand feet, yet I'm also enjoying a sensation I never dreamed possible. Everything is this moment. I'm flying, literally, for the first time in my life.

Actually, I'm diving. Or falling. With the pull of a cord I'm floating. The guy strapped to my back lets me know this is jump number 3,781. I believe him; no one that precise would lie. I ask if he ever gets tired of it. No way. Each and every one is like the first.

That mental state, being so consumed in the moment that space and time disappear, is not limited to skydiving. While I achieved it flying through the atmosphere, the situation does not need to be novel. If you want to get into the state known as flow, Hungarian psychologist Mihaly Csíkszentmihályi, the man behind the term, says the more you practice for it, the more likely you are to achieve it.

YOUR LOSS IS YOUR GAIN

In flow states, our sense of self-consciousness disappears. Sometimes time expands, at others it stops completely. Historically this experience has been called mystical, a peak experience, super-consciousness, spiritual, sacred, divine. Your sense of self dissolves. You're bigger than the cosmos, yet there's no "you" even there. It would feel disorienting if it didn't feel so *right*. You're in the pocket, you're on fire, you're in the zone; nothing can stop you.

Since many ways to enter this unique psychological state exist, Csíkszentmihályi conducted a large-scale global happiness survey to uncover what it entails. He asked people about the moments in life when they perform their best. He talked to Detroit assembly line workers and Japanese teenage motorcycle gang members, elderly Korean women, Navajo sheepherders, professional dancers, expert neurosurgeons, athletes, musicians, and many more. Everybody said that in flow states there's liquidity in their actions. Each decision blends seamlessly with the next. Genuine satisfaction occurs. This is especially true when creative abilities are expressed. This led Csíkszentmihályi to realize happiness doesn't simply happen. He writes, "Happiness, in fact, is a condition that must be prepared for, cultivated, and defended privately by each person. People who learn to control inner experiences will be able to determine the quality of their lives, which is as close as any of us can come to being happy."[1]

While happiness is one term, Csíkszentmihályi also discusses the lack of contentment many feel in their lives. He believes that by preparing for flow states you feel more at ease in your body and become more fulfilled in life. According to him, ten factors help create flow. While many of these components may be present, it is not necessary to experience all of them, though it is a good checklist:

- Clear goals that are challenging but attainable
- Strong concentration and focused attention
- The activity is intrinsically rewarding
- Feelings of serenity; a loss of self-consciousness
- Timelessness
- Immediate feedback
- Knowing the task is achievable
- Feelings of personal control
- Lack of awareness of physical needs
- Complete focus on the activity itself

While these are examples of what being in a flow state entails, it is also defined by specific affective and attentional states, including:

- Motivation
- High energy
- Moments of total absorption and immersion

Anecdotes are essential to understanding flow states, but researchers decided to view what's going on inside the brain during such experiences through fMRI scans. What was once considered subjective is now understood to be objective—precise neural responses are witnessed across the board. The fact that flow is objective surprised many experts. Researchers previously assumed that the prefrontal cortex (PFC) was where flow is processed. The PFC is responsible for complex cognitive abilities such as planning ahead, evaluating rewards and time, suppressing urges, making moral decisions, learning from experience, reacting to instinctual emotions, and having a sense of one's self. Yet the PFC actually *shuts down* during flow, which is known as transient hypofrontality. This is why flow feels instinctual and automatic: your sense of self, the neural region that creates your identity, steps back. The dorsolateral prefrontal cortex, or your "inner critic"[2] (also known as that nagging voice that says, "you can't do this"), is deactivated. This deactivation imbues you with a superhuman sense of courage. The thinking brain shuts down as the primitive, primary instinctual brain takes over. It's no wonder you feel a part of everything around you—the "you" *has* disappeared, or, at the very least, is taking a break.

The flow state is not just a shutdown. It actually occurs as the result of a synchronization of attentional and reward networks thanks to the balance of challenge and skill. Researchers are even able to artificially induce flow states in controlled environments by using transcranial direct-current stimulation (tDCS) to turn off the prefrontal cortex, allowing people to perform and learn more efficiently. Remember the scene in *The Matrix* where information is uploaded directly into Neo's brain? We're not there, but researchers are finding novel ways of influencing neurochemistry.

One eye-opening example involves a study conducted by DARPA, the Department of Defense's research division. Using video game imagery from a training platform that helps soldiers identify sniper rifles in hidden locations, those who had doses of tDCS learned the material twice as quickly as the group that received a sham dose.[3] If you consider how stressful seeking out these signals in foreign territories must be, an ability to both focus better and remain calm during high-stress situations is one incredible application of a deactivated PFC. The applications for such a mental and emotional state go far beyond the rigors of warfare, relevant to all of us regardless of what we do in life. Doing it to the best of our ability and, perhaps of equal importance, enjoying what we do, is something we can all appreciate. So let's dive a bit deeper into what flow entails.

HIERARCHY OF NEEDS

Look, there's dopamine again. Norepinephrine too. Endorphins, serotonin, and anandamide—that's a fatty acid neurotransmitter whose name is derived from the Sanskrit *ananda*, which means "bliss"—are all indicative of flow states. The PFC might be on vacation, but the brain is steadily serving a pleasant cocktail while you glide through your activity. Runners have their own term for it: runner's high. What would you call a bookworm's paradise? I suppose a reader's high will do, as flow states are applicable to those of us who love literature. In high school I served as my business class's accountant, falling in love with the act of adding up rows and columns. During my earliest years math was my favorite subject. That changed over the years, but the entranced state I entered while working on spreadsheets was certainly an accounting high.

You'll most hear about flow from extreme adventurers and professional athletes, though physical activity is not necessary. Flow is a transformation of the psychological realm open to anyone, anywhere, provided that certain conditions are met. A variety of triggers can bring about this state, including:

- Psychological triggers acting as internal activators to drive attention into the present moment. Deep focus. No multi-tasking; long periods of concentration on one task. Having a goal. One must know what they are doing and why they are doing it. When goals are clear, the mind has little room to wander.
- Environmental triggers are qualities in the immediate environment that bring individuals into flow. Risk and danger are important keys to unlocking flow because survival is fundamental to any organism. The brain's first priority is to focus on staying safe from any threat. An elevated sense of threat can actually enhance flow.

- Novelty, unpredictability, and complexity in an environment bring about flow in a similar way as risk. If we don't know what is happening next we pay close attention, especially if we are concerned.
- Social triggers occur when individuals share a goal. This balancing act provides enough focus and a shared solution, though one open to interpretation and challenging enough for creativity to exist. Potential for failure must exist for group flow to take place. In group flow the goal is the momentum, togetherness, and innovation that comes from amplifying one another's ideas and actions.

While we've been discussing individual flow, group flow is a phenomenon often witnessed in team sports. A group of individuals merge to form one unit. In the next chapter we'll see how musicians playing together trigger a similar neurochemistry, which creates its own flow. Whether alone or with others, creativity triggers flow while flow enhances creativity. Problem-solving is a great way to engage in flow activities, which is why my early love for math probably thrust me into such a deep sense of focus and purpose.

Having a sense of purpose is critical for our mental and emotional health. According to the Association for Psychological Science, living a purposeful life might help you live longer.[4] Nearly half a century before Csíkszentmihályi was developing his theory of flow, American psychologist Abraham Maslow created his hierarchy of needs, otherwise known as peak experiences. These are roadmaps to self-actualization. In his 1943 paper, "A Theory of Human Motivation" (and subsequent book *Motivation and Personality*), he introduced them, definable by three characteristics:

- Significance: The experience leads to an increased awareness of one's own life, which could become a turning point.
- Fulfillment: These experiences are intrinsically rewarding and generate positive emotions.
- Spiritual: During the experience one feels at peace with the world and loses track of time.

Maslow described these experiences as moments of rapture, ecstatic points where everything seems to fall perfectly into place.

One has a sense of ease and trust about their existence. This could involve falling in love or hearing new music that immediately captures you. Like Csíkszentmihályi, Maslow believed you could prepare for them. Self-actualizing people were likely to have them most often.

His hierarchy of needs is essentially a ladder, with self-actualizing people at the highest rung. While Maslow includes a spiritual element, self-actualizing implies that this particular psychological state is attainable by anyone whose basic mental and emotional needs are met. People actively striving to reach their greatest potential are the most successful climbers. As with flow states, peak experiences mean having greater focus while losing a sense of self-consciousness. Some qualities of these climbers include playfulness, effortlessness, self-sufficiency, wholeness, and aliveness. They wake up in the morning looking forward to the day ahead and go to sleep feeling accomplished.

This seems like such a basic concept, yet Csíkszentmihályi recognized that the biggest stumbling block is our hubris. "The primary reason it is so difficult to achieve happiness," he writes, "centers on the fact that, contrary to the myths mankind has developed to reassure itself, the universe was not created to answer our needs."[5] Frustration is a necessary component of existence, not an aberration. This harkens back to Buddha, the sage who recognized we suffer because we do not view the world correctly. We think the universe is here to serve our needs; suffering occurs when we recognize that it does not. The conflict resides within our own mind, not with the true functioning of nature, of which we know very little. Our brain might be designed for storytelling, but that does not mean the randomness of the universe has a narrative. That we desire it to have one is faulty perception. Stories serve an important purpose in binding humans together to work against the elements and forces of nature. To believe the planet has a duty to cater to our stories, according to Buddha and Csíkszentmihályi and many others, is where the problems begin.

Austrian psychiatrist Viktor Frankl had a similar take. The founder of logotherapy recognized that the insistent drive toward success was part of what held people back. For Csíkszentmihályi, having clear goals and attainable ambitions is important, but in a sense the goal is almost secondary to the process. Frankl believed the responsibility of each human is to live up to the challenges at hand and not only contemplate the results—a theory born after surviving the Holocaust. The loss of self-consciousness that Csíkszentmihályi dubbed flow took on a broader social meaning in Frankl's eyes. "Don't aim at success—the more you aim at it and make it a target, the more you are going to miss it. For success, like happiness, cannot be pursued; it must ensue . . . as the unintended side-effect of one's personal dedication to a course greater than oneself."[6]

This requires diving deeply inside an interior landscape not necessarily filled with joy and pleasure. Perhaps the most famous of mythologist Joseph Campbell's sayings is "follow your bliss." True, it sounds quite lovely. Who wouldn't want to exist in a state of relentless ecstasy? Now let's read his quote in full. It's a reminder that self-actualizing has never been easy, but the rewards—sense of awareness and ease of body; attaining a mindset of the perceptual moment—are extremely valuable. Campbell says the first step is recognizing the pain entwined with bliss. He continues, "The best thing I can say is to follow your bliss. If your bliss is just your fun and your excitement, you're on the wrong track. I mean, you need instruction. Know where your bliss is. And that involves coming down to a deep place in yourself."[7]

WISDOM OVER WEALTH

How does one practice for such a state, as Csíkszentmihályi suggests? In this book we've discussed physical training in terms of exercise and mental training in yoga and meditation. Emotional training is implicated in all of these formats. The real field of play is life, however. I often remind my yoga students that the studio we're practicing in is a preparation for what happens when we leave the room. How you respond to your physical practice is most likely indicative of how you react when faced with challenges in life. Do you laugh it off or get angry when falling out of a balancing posture? Are you jealous of the woman next to you rocking an arm balance while you can't get a handle on your mat given the amount of sweat that's accumulated? Or do you do your best with what you have, knowing that the process is more important than the goal, as Frankl believes?

It all comes back to mindset. The yoga studio is a relatively safe space to work through issues, gain strength and resilience, and hopefully find a little bit of inner peace. Life isn't always so safe, but the rules don't necessarily change. An ability to persevere despite obstacles and setbacks is an admirable quality. This transcends any physical posture and offers a bit of insight into succeeding at life. It also helps you enjoy it as well.

While there are a variety of conditions that lead to flow, the following are in alignment with Csíkszentmihályi's recommendations.

- You have a chance of completing the task at hand.
- You must be able to concentrate on what you're doing.
- The task has clear goals and provides immediate feedback.
- You act with a deep but effortless involvement while removing the worries and frustrations of everyday life.
- Enjoyable experiences allow you to exercise a sense of control over your actions.
- Concern for the self disappears, yet your sense of self emerges stronger after the experience is over.
- Your sense of time is altered; hours pass by in minutes while minutes seem like hours.

The paradox is that you lose control while gaining mastery. It's only your sense of self, which is a construct to begin with, that is loosened, just as it is in sleep. In fact, recent research shows that you can develop motor skills via lucid dreaming as effectively as practicing the same skill while awake.[8] Consciousness is but a sliver of the mechanisms we use to navigate our environment. While it's ultimately essential for many of the pleasures we enjoy, it is not always the best guide, given the unnecessary fears and worries we get bogged down in. Letting loose of control in an enjoyable activity is some of the most potent medicine available for our well-being—no prescription needed, always on hand when you're ready to take it.

In *Born to Run*, Christopher McDougall writes about an unintended consequence that occurred when companies started sponsoring runners: their times got worse.[9] He suggests that Americans get it backwards, because of the following belief: acquire wealth and then wisdom (or happiness, as it often goes) will come. Runners that began worrying about times and winning stopped enjoying running; the very skill they were trying to improve took a hit due to obsessing over the wrong aspects. Like running, practicing gratitude is one powerful step in enjoying this very moment you're in.

Another involves what I consider the greatest auditory contribution to our species ever. What gets me into flow more than anything else is listening to music. As it turns out, it's a skill we can all enjoy.

Chapter 12

The Perfect Soundtrack

"All of us have had the experience of being transported by the sheer beauty of music—suddenly finding ourselves in tears, not knowing whether they are of joy or sadness, suddenly feeling a sense of the sublime, or a great stillness within."

—Oliver Sacks, *Brain: A Journal of Neurology*

SONIC ANIMALS

Music only exists inside of your head. Single notes travel through the air, causing your eardrums to vibrate, though it isn't only that canal informing your brain that something special is going down. Sound waves hit your eardrum, quickly transferred to the cochlea in your inner ear where microscopic hair cells dance. This movement turns the mechanical energy of the wave into chemical signals that stimulate auditory nerves to fire action potentials. From here music travels to your primary auditory cortex in the temporal lobe, and then through your primary processing system, the primitive emotional area of your brain. You also *feel* music through your skin. These disparate noises are transformed into nerve impulses where the elements—pitch, melody, timbre, rhythm—combine to form the patterns called *music*. Your brain processes these random snippets of sound into one of the most meaningful aspects of being human.

Songs have defined people and places throughout history. *What* music you enjoy is dictated by personal tastes, culture, timing, and just plain luck; *that* music is essential is rarely debated. Pythagoras postulated that the cosmos is strung together by a string of notes conspiring to create an elegant symphony. While today we can actually hear the sounds of space—I doubt it'll make your next playlist—we can dream that Pythagoras was right when staring into the starry sky.

I recall the soundtrack of the rainy New Brunswick morning when my heart was first broken. Jeff Buckley's mournful "Lover, You Should've Come Over" remains closer to me than the smell of the cigarette she was smoking or what we wore. As a certified fourteen-year-old rock-and-roll fan I'll never forget riding my bike to Borough Park to play street hockey as my best friend, Andrew, pumped Public Enemy's "Fight the Power" on his fake ghetto blaster. Ever since has my head bounced to hip-hop. Nor will I fail to remember driving through Texas pumping The Roots' "Don't Feel Right," as the minivan's puny speakers sputtered while attempting to register the bass, nor the opening drum beat of "The Things That I Used to Do" during a college trip to Lowell, Massachusetts to meet Allen Ginsberg with eight guys packed tightly inside of one midsize sedan. Music defines time as well as people and places.

We all have soundtracks to life. As I reminisce over mine you might be recalling your own. And music remains with us for life. People suffering from dementia might not be able to recall that their husband visited yesterday, but they can often tell if you play a wrong note in a song they haven't heard for sixty years. Some Parkinson's disease patients that otherwise cannot walk are able to stand up and dance when certain music is played; some autistic children respond better to music than any other form of therapy.

Music is not only therapeutic for people suffering from a disease. It releases dopamine in our striatum, an ancient neural reward system—music gives us the same pleasure as food, sex, and drugs. Musicians sometimes turn to cocaine and amphetamines because performing results in similar neurochemistry. For fitness junkies, listening to music increases pain threshold and endurance.

Complex music helps us learn better. As a symphony slowly builds, myriad neural regions work in conjunction to relate the sounds to our bodies. Interestingly, the same can be said for complex movements, which is why music is such an important component in fitness.

That movement and music are connected should not surprise us. Historically, many cultures used the same word for "dance" and "song." How to effectively use music for movement is another story. We know we love music, and we know the music we love, but how to use it in the context of movement is an art form itself.

More Than a Feeling

I've taken numerous classes in which the instructor plays the wrong music. I'm not talking about music I don't like. That is a subjective preference dependent upon culture, environment, exposure, and taste. The teacher was playing a rhythm that contradicted what they were asking me to perform with my body.

Music affects us subconsciously. There's a soundtrack for restaurants that want you to leave quickly; there's a formula in department stores asking you to linger (and shop more). Hollywood music directors know how to strike emotional chords. Watch the most dramatic scenes in cinematic history without music and everything falls apart. There's even an imperceptible tone used in horror films. You can't hear the tension building, but your body certainly feels it.

This is why music is so important in fitness. I once took a yoga class in which the instructor played the same electronic opera song for a half-hour. Then he switched to a Peruvian pan flute record that opened with a cover of "Hotel California." Besides the obvious nightmare of such an aesthetic, the throbbing drum 'n bass rhythm was completely at odds with holding postures for a minute. A rhythm of 160-plus beats per minute (BPM) forces your body to move; static postures are not a movement equivalent to this tempo. To switch from the intense rush of an auditory assault to a downtempo beat is jarring. There's no story being told, at least not one any sane body would want to tell.

The same has been the case the few times I've taken yoga classes where the teacher plays hip-hop during *Savasana*, the resting "corpse pose" at the end of class. The goal of this pose is to physiologically slow down the body as much as possible; it is parasympathetic mode personified. Playing rap instead of ambient music during this critical healing period is a double dose of wrong. Your brain entrains to beats whether or not you want it to. Even though hip-hop beats are generally slower than house (generally 80 BPM compared to 120 BPM), the genre uses a strong kick drum and bass, causing your motor neurons to prepare for action. Your breathing rate increases when you should be steadily floating along.

Another issue is lyrics. There are two main language centers in your brain: Wernicke's area and Broca's area. The latter helps you to speak and form sentences. Wernicke's allows you to understand written and spoken language. It's difficult to relax when your brain is translating a song's narrative. Further, parasympathetic mode involves staying present, one of the keystones of yoga. When you start contemplating the lyrics, chances are you'll relate them to your life. This pulls you from the moment, the very intention of *Savasana*.

Narrative is important, though it doesn't necessarily require language. Music is older than fables and mythologies. Language is a way of communicating ideas—grunts, sighs, facial expressions, and pantomimes are all systems of communication. Your brain is wired for storytelling. The best instructors tell epic tales every time they step in front of a class. Postures, lights, heat, environment, and music are all important characters in this sweaty drama. Top teachers are masterful conductors stringing these pieces together. Those who do not take group classes can control these elements for your own ritualistic experience. Music is of primary importance in this.

When I began teaching yoga, I recalled mythologist Joseph Campbell's four stages of storytelling. Every class I've taught since, be it yoga or another discipline, has intentionally followed this trajectory. Campbell realized that stories from various unrelated cultures repeated the same motifs in a similar order. This sequence can be found throughout literature and cinema—Hollywood blockbusters rely on it as much as novels do. We spend one-third of our waking hours telling ourselves stories thanks to our imagination.[1] There is something primal about this narrative arc, making it a perfect template for fitness routines and their soundtracks.

- **Setting Off.** Mythologies begin on rocky turf: a trauma, disaster, or inner call sparks the hero's inquisitiveness. Think Luke Skywalker. (George Lucas met with Campbell to discuss mythological motifs.) Skywalker dreamed of becoming a rebel alliance pilot, but would never have acted had stormtroopers not murdered his aunt and uncle. This traumatic event kicked off the entire series (well, in the order presented by Lucas). In fitness, everyone has a goal, be it emotional, physical, or spiritual. This goal does not even have to be direct: In the chivalry tales of the Arthurian cycles, a knight always sets off on a quest in the darkest part of the forest where no trail has been carved. He must blaze a new trail. The setting off, or "warm-up" in fitness terms, prepares you for the journey ahead. Musically, this is a perfect opportunity for strings, midtempo beats, or any music that builds in momentum and features an element of seeking, of stoking excitement as you step onto the road.
- **The Journey.** Now the action happens: the yoga flow, the high intensity of HIIT, the heart of a trail run. Heat is built, strength gained, focus honed. Think of Rama's search for Sita in the *Ramayana*, or Galahad's epic quest attaining the Holy Grail. You're challenged physically and mentally; the music is at its most upbeat and fluid. Throbbing house music, heady hip-hop, Afrobeat, upbeat soul. This is also where your mind is most engaged on movement, offering you a perfect opportunity to be your most creative, physically and musically.
- **The Return.** In every mythology the hero must return home, like Gilgamesh after finding the secret of everlasting life (a plant that ended up in a fish's mouth, much to the king's chagrin). In psychological terms, this is integration; in trauma, recovering from a wound. Physically, this is correlated to stretching after an intense bout of exercise, offering you an opportunity to enter a meditative space. Downtempo beats and ambient music is

perfect for this cooldown phase. Lyrical ballads also work, especially if inspiring. As you move from sympathetic to parasympathetic mode, a little storytelling sets the tone nicely.

- **Integration.** Otherwise known as regeneration. The quest is over as the hero steps into the next phase of life. A lesson has been learned; the hero must now integrate that knowledge into his or her new life. Meditation, deep static stretching, foam rolling, mysofascial release, Feldenkrais techniques, and complete relaxation take you into a deeply personal space to recharge. Ambient, instrumental, and some classical music are perfect for this phase. While the efficacy of binaural beats—two pure-tone sine waves playing simultaneously that create an illusion of a third tone; they are thought to enhance focus and relaxation—is debated, I've personally had great success with them. As there is not a ton of evidence in the literature of their exact role in our brain, I'll leave it to you to try out. There are plenty of apps that offer biurnal beats if you are inclined to try. Whatever you choose, this phase should be reflected by the chillest sounds in your library.

Like creating a workout, designing playlists takes time. I began making cassette mixtapes in the eighties and have never slowed down. One of the fortunate aspects of music services like Spotify is how easy it is to not only make them, but share them publicly—a boon if you're seeking inspiration for workouts. (I maintain weekly yoga, fitness, and studio cycling playlists, as well as offer yoga and house mixtapes, on my personal website, derekberes.com.)

Storytelling is the larger narrative of music and fitness. We don't necessarily need to know the science behind music to recognize if the soundtrack feels right. As I kept taking classes that didn't sync up, though, I wondered why that is. For the rest of this chapter we'll explore how much music affects our brain. The sheer amount of material could be a separate book, as I spent over two years developing Flow Play, a music, yoga, and neuroscience program at Equinox Fitness, alongside my colleague Philip Steir. I've decided to just include some of my favorite studies with the hopes that they empower you in making great playlists and movement sessions for yourself and your students.

SOUNDTRACK FOR LIFE

So much of this book has been about cultivating an ability to pay attention, a fundamental cognitive process upon which more complex ones rely. To learn new movement patterns—say, riding a bike—you have to devote your full mental resources to the task at hand. Though conscious processes become unconscious over time, you're constantly being challenged to prevent an intrusion of distracting information. Music is one insightful means by which scientists are learning about attention. A team at Stanford University scanned subjects who were listening to an eighteenth-century composer in hopes of better understanding how the human brain makes sense of the world.[2] Music directly engages neural regions responsible for attention and in prediction-making. Interestingly, peak activity occurred during the silence between musical movements, as if the brain is anticipating what's going to happen next, reminding us once again of Rodolfo Llinás's philosophy that movement is the art of prediction.

Selective attention is the ability to focus on a task while ignoring competing stimuli—writing a book while paying no mind to email dings or Facebook posts, for example. The Stanford team found that music helps the brain organize information in exactly this way through a process known as "event segmentation." Your brain is able to partition meaningful information into a narrative that makes sense, filtering out irrelevant data. This is one of the most important facets of consciousness: removing the overwhelming amount of information you receive every day to focus on what really matters. Music primes your brain to sustain relevant data and make better predictions.

Your brain is always predicting music. Rarely is it a fan of abstract sounds; formulaic pop and dance music work for a reason. You know the beat is about to drop or a melody chime in even if it's your first time hearing a song. In this way music exploits your brain's evolutionary reward system, as it releases dopamine several seconds *before* the beat actually drops, during what's called the anticipation phase. Merely preparing for the pleasure of the beat is its own reward.

This is not relegated to music alone; businesses are constantly taking advantage of this evolutionary feature. For example, my first job in New York City was as a crossword puzzle editor. The magazine I worked for required that the predominant number of puzzles in each magazine be easy, meaning I had to repeat the same clues for the same words issue after issue. (Two people create a crossword puzzle. The designer constructs the grid and fills in the words, and the editor invents the clues.) This magazine is a top-seller because people feel a sense of satisfaction every issue, ensuring that they'll buy another next month. Music exploits this same system, so long as the beat drops. Ever take a class in which the power suddenly shuts off during a peak emotional moment? Or worse, the instructor just shuts off a song without fading it? They might believe it's no big deal. Your nervous system does not agree.

Anticipation helps you focus as your brain prepares for the next movement or sequence. We all know the value of music in fitness classes. But this works in your career as well. University of Miami associate professor Teresa Lesiuk discovered that workers listening to music in creative jobs, such as software designers and information technology specialists, complete tasks quicker and create better ideas than those working in silence. From her research it appears that music improves their mood as well as focus. She also realized that music helps calm workers during stressful situations, as it delays emotional reactivity. People who listen to music while on the job make less hasty decisions.[3]

Style matters. The key is choosing music that calms the primitive part of your brain while allowing for greater focus than during silence. Ideal music should occupy your brain just enough to help focus. Music with emotional or sentimental overtones is likely to stimulate your amygdala, the brain's emotional processing center, and hippocampus, the weigh station for memories, in your limbic emotional system. If the songs are too fast, variable, or loud, your locus coeruleus, a region that responds to stress and panic, jumps into action. Turn down the dubstep; turn up Cinematic Orchestra.

Your playlist should lean toward that band's instrumentals if focus is your goal, however. As mentioned, music with lyrics is distracting when compared to those with instruments alone, which is why film scores generally do not have lyrics. Music in the range of sixty to ninety BPM decreases neural activity, making downtempo beats ideal for work time. This tempo leads to relaxed, though aware, alpha states in your brain, with a decrease in higher activity beta waves.[4] Alpha wave increases promote a sense of timelessness, motivation, and decreased self-awareness—flow states. By helping boost focus and dissuade distraction, music is a wonderful tool for dropping into the present moment.

Presence is a word shrouded in ambiguity, but researchers do have a working definition. Presence is grounded in time, and time is a relatable phenomena—it arises during your nervous system's perception of an interaction with the world. The present moment is the minimum amount of time it takes to sense and perceive and categorize, which is dictated by the speed at which your neurons fire. Psychologists label this the "perceptual present." When you focus on music, this mental state is readily attainable. Ironically, being present in time usually results in not feeling time. There's truth in the saying "lost in the music," though in some ways you find something valuable during these moments. Music is a form of meditation for both players and listeners. For that we once again thank chemistry.

TIME TO GET HIGH

Oxytocin is a social drug. The physiological effects of this hormone are staggering. It is most famously known for its role in inducing labor and post-orgasmic cooldown. It also modulates inflammation, increases trust and empathy, inspires learning and memory, bonds mother with child, reduces social anxiety, and, according to some studies, may play a role in inhibiting the production of cortisol and could even help quiet autism's repetitive behaviors. Like all hormones, its role is not entirely angelic: there is evidence that it negatively affects certain social behaviors.[5] But there's no doubt we want regular doses of this hormone.

Music provides it. When people play music together, oxytocin is released.[6] Throughout our evolutionary history, music has united people and allowed communities to feel less anxious and more trusting. It binds groups together in times of trial and warfare and is the glue that holds people together in all walks of life. English psychoanalyst Anthony Storr specialized in music and mental states. He writes, "In all societies, a primary function of music is collective and communal, to bring and bind people together. People sing together, dance together, in every culture, and one can imagine them doing so, around the first fires, a hundred thousand years ago."[7]

The origins of music are unknown, but many researchers speculate that music played an essential role in social interaction, providing a vehicle for building trust with others. Vocal music may have originated as a communication tool to relate to other tribe members, even strangers. Historically, most cultures gave birth to traveling bards journeying from place to place relating the social issues of the day. In Africa, the *griot* tradition has remained in families for centuries, as have the *qawwali* lineages of Pakistan, which precede the founding of that country by at least six hundred years. American folk music has played an important role in the formation and maintenance of entire societies, just as woodwind and drum music has been a force for Native American heritage. We trust music in the same manner that we trust the sounds in nature: to communicate what is taking place in our environment. When we hear thunder we know a storm is coming. When we hear birds chirping we know the weather is favorable. When we hear anger in a predator's vocal expression it's time to leave, quickly. We trust music to let us weep, feel ecstasy, give us strength, fuel our confidence, exercise harder and longer, focus more efficiently, and experience the power of romantic love. Music does this by mimicking our brain system perfectly. Music that we love triggers the same area of the brain that makes romantic love feel amazing. Trust and music go hand in hand; both have the ability to transform our existence by altering our brain's chemical state. Oxytocin changes how we navigate, behave, and make decisions. Music is a primary driver of this change.

And music is healing—not only metaphorically. One study showed that music helped boost patients' oxytocin levels while reducing anxiety after heart surgery, both of which aided the healing process.[8] Music has been shown to improve cognitive abilities in children with learning disabilities, help elderly people feel more connected to the world, and help those who were nearly crippled to physically move again. The therapeutic aspects of music even help a badly damaged brain renew itself. That's right: music aids in regeneration.

To take a famous example, Arizona politician Gabrielle Giffords survived a shooting spree that killed six and injured a dozen others. Her coma-inducing gunshot wound to the left hemisphere of her brain left her unable to speak, but the damage has in part been repaired through music. Her music therapist notes that Giffords responds well to music because "she knows a lot of songs."[9] Through repetition of singing, her speech and memory functions, as well as other higher cognitive processes, returned. Therapies like music speech stimulation and melodic intonation therapy help patients with damage to the brain's communication center learn to speak again.

Music also renews the brain by creating new neural pathways. When language and speaking skills are no longer effective, therapists have patients sing to build a new pathway for speech. Evidence that music plays an important role in recovering from brain injuries is growing. The way music activates the brain and exhibits energizing effects is helping neuroscientists and researchers find ways to advance neuroplasticity and create new therapies to help heal neurological disease and injury. Music is linked to brain areas that control memory, emotions, and movement. It triggers the brain's primitive emotional areas first—emotions that feel instinctual and automatic are part of our ancient brain system. The body naturally aligns with a rhythm in the environment and translates the rhythm as movement while activating the motor cortex.

All adult mammals, humans included, have a limited ability to replace brain cells after they are lost to disease or injury. Scientists turned to the songbird to understand how learning and memory may help heal brain damage in a similar manner as they did for Giffords. Juvenile songbirds are able to regenerate multitudes of neurons every year. Scientists are attempting to decode the genetic programs behind this incredible capability in order to help replace the neurons lost in human brains by Alzheimer's, Parkinson's, stroke, and paralysis. While we enjoy birdsongs, these animals do not emerge from the egg singing; they learn by listening, just like humans do. As they practice, their brain's "song center" greatly increases the number and activity of neurons. Once born, these cells migrate throughout the brain, finding connections with established neurons in much the same way that BDNF becomes a system-wide fertilizer. While this also happens in humans, the rate at which it occurs in songbirds is astounding. This research provides valuable clues to not only understanding the genetic mechanisms behind the process of neural regeneration but how music, rhythm, melodies, and listening aid in memory development and learning. Researchers hope this will help create music-driven stem cell-based therapies for cell loss and brain damage in humans.

Moving beyond neural regeneration, music has been implicated in physical therapy as well. For people who've sustained injuries, the use of rhythmic patterns, whether from a metronome or music, aids in prolonging exercise in rehabilitative therapy. Thanks to the brain's ability to entrain to a beat, it is already helping Parkinson's patients move to a rhythm, whereas they could not control their motions otherwise.[10] This is also why oftentimes you cannot control your fingers when a beat comes on. With your motor neurons fired, movement is impossible to ignore.

Certain music inspires movement; others whisk us into parasympathetic mode. Importantly, our automatic relaxation response includes the reduction of anxiety and stress, another aspect of music's healing effects. Music allows patients to use less pain medication when listening to enjoyable or relaxing music. This autonomic relaxation response impacts our hormone and immune responses as well.

Besides the release of dopamine, serotonin, and natural opiates that the body produces when affected by music, a measurable decrease in cortisol is one of music's greatest triumphs over our nervous system. As noted earlier, sustained levels of cortisol prematurely kill us, making music therapy important for us on a number of critical levels.

The relaxation response changes our brain's electromagnetic waveforms. When brainwaves move from one state, such as alpha waves, or relaxed wakefulness, to theta, or deep relaxation, it affects the rhythm of our heart and breath as well. Music influences the electrochemical activity by releasing certain neurotransmitters that fire and pulse. We then relax. When tempos are at a slower rate of sixty BPM, the song matches the relaxed heartbeat, calming the brain and breath. Deep breathing to a slow tempo induces muscle relaxation while increasing focus. Not only does downtempo and ambient music reduce anxiety, but it helps you train your mind to stay calm and collected in the face of life's difficulties. Over time this sort of deep listening helps you transform your "monkey mind" to one that is grounded, calm, and focused. That is also why music is believed to have a spiritual purpose.

INNER JUKEBOX

I spent countless hours during my youth listening to 89.5 FM, Seton Hall's college radio station. While going through the regular dose of teenage trials and angst, the magic of closing my door, lying on my bedroom floor, and tuning in to hours of indie rock transported me to a place removed in space and time from my suburban upbringing. Like many children of the eighties I had a Walkman, then a Discman, briefly carried a mini-disc player, and ultimately graduated to an iPod until my phone handled all necessary duties. Even today, my phone is little more than a music and podcast player. During that entire evolution of devices, what's been consistent are headphones and long walks. This book might be about changing habits, but some need no improvement.

Years ago a friend of mine wore a shirt that read, "My God is Music." I'm not a religious person, but that might be the most meaningful sentiment I've come across regarding as elusive and pervasive an idea as divinity. There's good reason that music has been at the heart of ritual experiences throughout time. It requires the cooperation of more neural regions than anything else, syncing up those regions in what results in an ecstatic, emotional, and cathartic experience, carrying us deeply inside of ourselves. It is a personal and communal experience. Music moves us and we move with it.

According to neuroscientist Dan Levitin, music serves an evolutionary purpose as well as being a natural phenomenological expression of human spirituality.[11] Levitin believes music replicates empathy, trust, love, and the ability to be emotionally moved by something—essential components of spirituality. It binds us together and, when the conditions call for it, tears us apart with the march of a war song.

In many ways we create music during every step of life. We generate rhythm on a daily basis. The proper functioning of our brain, heart, and breath are necessary for mental, physical, and emotional health; each of these functions has its own rhythm upon which life depends. If that rhythm is thrown off slightly we are immediately aware. Organic pulses in nature create music as well: the rhythm of a river, a gust of wind.

But the way we consume music has changed drastically over the last century. As odd as it sounds now, hearing music detached from the musicians playing it is a phenomenon that began when affordable record players hit the market shortly after the Great Depression. Jazz and gospel, both spiritual, devotional forms of music, were the first widely marketed genres; classical, arguably another spiritual category, came in tow. Suddenly, humans could hear a song whenever they desired, completely restructuring an art form as old as any known system of communication. Like all technological advances, it's come at a cost.

Along with advances in music came damaging strides in noise. Humans flock to urban environments today, for good reason: we like connection. The trade-off is an assault of noise on our nervous systems. Background noise affects our bodies and minds in ways that many never consider. Workplace noise raises blood pressure, causes exhaustion, and increases negative attitudes. Physiological stress levels are elevated when hearing constant traffic, raising glucocorticoid enzyme levels that contribute to anxiety and stress by up to 40 percent. Excessive noise also damages learning in young children, and is considered the most negative environmental condition except for air pollution.[12]

Sadly, we create more noise than we realize in the most unsuspecting of places. When I moved to Los Angeles in 2011 I headed straight for the beach; five years and three apartments later I still live within a fifteen-minute drive. I conducted a fair amount of research for this book in my second office, with a towel laid out twenty feet from the waves, my favorite music of all. So when I come across people blasting music through their tinny phone speakers on the beach I feel like I've run straight into a microcosm of our social disconnection: the inability to appreciate the music of nature. I've also come across trail runners, earbuds stuffed into cranium, unaware that I'm trying to pass—a more dangerous carnivore would quickly have its way. Some even climb hills with their phone strapped to their belt, podcast voices replacing the sound of chirps, wind, and leaves. This desire for nature is more than a personal preference. It's a tragedy that we've grown so distant from her.

Technology has given us so much, but it's taken away just as much. This is the focus of the last chapter. The inability to separate modes—the reality in front of us versus a reality removed in time and space, which is much of what digital and wireless technologies offer—is at the root of many health issues, from mismatch diseases and diseases of affluence to mental health disorders such as depression and anxiety. These problems are solvable, but knowing how to use our devices without becoming used by them is the first step in that direction. Given the addictive patterns many technologies create in our neurochemistry, fostering a very real emotional and mental dependence, combined with the vested interest that companies have in keeping you addicted, this is perhaps the hardest step of our entire journey together. But, as I'll argue, this one step helps make all of the others we've discussed that much easier. When you learn to control your attention, you can attend to whatever you're focused on.

Music is no cure-all. I will, however, gladly enjoy the fruits of technology in this regard. A century ago I'd have to buy a ticket to hear Massive Attack, my soundtrack while writing much of this chapter. The midtempo beats, the wide range of guest vocalists, warm bass tones, and ambient strings have been creative fuel for contemplating my favorite art. Perhaps that's music's greatest offering: a friend that's always there when you need it. Growing up I didn't understand the chemistry occurring in my brain and blood as I drifted to unimaginable realms that helped me deal with the one I had to face every day. It didn't matter—it helped tremendously. Knowing what type of music aids in the various physical workouts, from HIIT to meditation, now serves to deepen my experience. For the last leg of our travels together, we tune into what's directly in front of us. As much as the past and future offer, this moment now matters most.

Chapter 13

Attention, Please

"In solving problems, technology creates new problems, and we seem, as in *Through the Looking Glass,* to have to keep running faster and faster to stay where we are. The question is then whether technical progress actually 'gets anywhere' in the sense of increasing the delight and happiness of life."

—Alan Watts, *The Book*

Inside the Glass Cage

Children do not like basements. They're subterranean realms where creatures live. When you descend the stairs, the temperature drops; the chill then ascends as your feet touch the unfinished floor. Our downstairs was often used, however, since it housed the washing machine, pool table, and my father's workbench and gym. Next to the weights lived a desk wedged between a bathroom and pantry. On top of the desks sat a Commodore VIC-20, the first personal computer to ever sell a million units.

My father began working in computer operations in the sixties. For my whole life, I always had a keyboard and monitor to learn programs and play games on. My earliest memory of it involved hours tapping keys during Blitz, a Tetris-like strategy game in which you had to knock down buildings as a pixelated plane scrolled line by line. Preempting a national tragedy, the only way the game ended was replicated in downtown Manhattan just over two decades after its 1979 release.

The basement is a perfect metaphor for technology's place in my life at that early age: somewhere you retreated on occasion, when it was too cold or too late to be outside, to get lost in a rush of imagery and develop problem-solving skills. Floppy disks were laborious; waiting for five kilobytes of information to load took minutes. The computer was dessert when your body was tired from a day of wiffleball, bike riding, and swimming. You didn't worry much about the screen's effects on your visual system because you simply didn't spend enough time staring at one for it to be of concern.

How times have changed.

My next train of thought is to claim that I'm no Luddite, but that wouldn't be fair to that movement. While the word is generally used to represent anyone against technology, the nineteenth-century English social rebellion is an apt comparison to problems we face today. During the second decade of that century, textile workers raged against factory owners that were implementing machines to cut labor costs, which meant they didn't have to hire as many laborers. Workers mobilized to fight the mechanization of skilled work that required human touch and ingenuity. Over the next century the British government and its police were often called to put down strikes and punish irate workers who were smashing machinery. These men were not necessarily against technology; they were fighting for survival.

The promises of machinery were too seductive for business owners to deny. An automated world saved them money, ensured efficiency, and lowered overhead. In *The Glass Cage*, Nicholas Carr discusses "automation addiction," using the airline industry as a lens to study this concept. Modern pilots are required to perform roughly three to four minutes of manual labor during a flight thanks to automated navigational technologies. Their attention is required during the entire flight, however, inputting data and ensuring the plane stays on course. There are two problems with this, Carr writes. First off, technology isn't infallible, especially when it comes to hurling hundreds of people thirty-five thousand feet off the ground.

Minor infractions in weather and gear can, at any moment, take the entire system offline, much like a small cut on your foot can lead to a life-threatening infection if not attended to. This leads to the second problem: when something does go offline, the pilots' cognitive skills are challenged in ways they're unaccustomed to, given that they spend most of their time *not* handling the plane. A few recent crashes, some small, some not so, are attributed to the pilot not knowing what to do (or doing the exact opposite of what they should be doing) when technology goes awry.

"We become so confident that the machine will work flawlessly," Carr writes, "handling any challenge that may arise, that we allow our attention to drift. We disengage from our work, or at least from the part of it that the software is handling, and as a result may miss signals that something is amiss."[1]

Carr discusses the importance of the "generation effect." When you force your brains to fill in a blank, you're more likely to remember what you're learning. For example, Carr uses *Hot: Cold*. When research participants were instead presented with *Hot: C*. They knew what the *C* represented. Since they had to fill in the blank, they retained the information better than when it was simply presented to them outright.[2] Interestingly, the process by which we learn is called automatization, which entails learning a procedural skill so that it becomes automatic and intuitive (tying a shoelace, riding a bike). Once the skill is second nature automaticity has been achieved. This is a good thing as our cognitive resources shift from a mundane task to higher thought processes. The problem with relying on technology is a deadening of the impulse to learn nuanced skills. We call computers intuitive, but when they don't respond exactly how we expect them to, or when we have to learn a new program that involves more than click-and-drag, impatience kicks in. There is a neurological reason for this: "Rather than extending the brain's innate capacity for automaticity, automation too often becomes an impediment to automatization. In relieving us of repetitive mental exercise, it also relieves us of deep learning."[3]

I'm writing this chapter over a weekend while I'm participating in a kettlebell certification course. During the opening session, our instructor informed us that he was not going to be talking much over the weekend. He feels we'll learn better if we have hands-on experience swinging the bells rather than over-explaining why and how to do it. And he's right. If you're familiar with kettlebells, swings are designed as a posterior-chain exercise, yet many people misinterpret the intention and treat them as an anterior-chain exercise; instead of hinging from the hips they squat and use their arms too much. Given how much squatting I do in yoga and VIPR it's very natural for me, while I reserve hip hinging for dead lifts. Since I rarely explode through a hinge pattern, my first few swings were squats. Our last task on day one was an intense ten-minute workout, involving ten sets of ten swings and ten push-ups with minimal breaks. By the time we began the swings felt natural and intuitive, which makes sense given that I'd spent half a day working on mechanics. No app was going to offer me that knowledge.

Mechanics of another sort is what caused Matthew B. Crawford to quit a lucrative job at a Washington DC think tank to fix motorcycles. Depression set in working in an office, as he was unable to use his body in the way it was designed by nature. Add in that it required him to contradict basic ethical beliefs to propel forward political agendas and his tenure was short-lived. Yet leaving a "prestigious" position to assume a job as a "lowly" mechanic opened his eyes to a bigger problem: those keeping society in working order—plumbers, mechanics, electricians, and construction workers—are necessary yet reviled. You rarely hear parents champion their children's future as laborers even though without such toil—without such creativity and hands-on experience—civilization could not exist. The "higher" realm of certain occupations, such as in finance and law, bolsters the automated world even as their work proves dangerous to the society fawning over them. The banking crisis of 2008, in which high-risk investments heavily relied on algorithms, did little to dissuade college graduates from seeking this line of work. The problems of automation and perception continue to worsen.

Crawford is skeptical of much of what automation promises. The "disburdening" provided by technological advance also removes from us personal responsibility. I once had a boss who would email me criticisms from her office, which was roughly ten feet from my own. The computer provided a screen in which she did not have to look me directly in the eyes. My response was always the same: I'd get up from my desk and walk those ten feet. While this befuddled her, it also kept potential tension from getting worse. When emotions and ideas are invisibly transported across time and space instead of physically moving your body to accomplish the same (and really, much more), there is too much room for misunderstanding—and expectations, as Crawford writes. "Consider the angry feeling that bubbles up in this person when, in a public bathroom, he finds himself waving his hands under the faucet, trying to elicit a few seconds of water from a futile rain dance of guessed-at mudras. This man would like to know: Why should there not be a *handle*? Instead he is asked to supplicate invisible powers."[4]

Crawford points out that an early usage of the word *liberal*, as in a liberal arts education, was used to distinguish the work of the "mind" from the "servile arts," occupations that require a little elbow grease. The liberal is free while the mechanic is a slave laborer, bound to the machine that is his sustenance. Yet, given all the information in this book so far, we can understand how ludicrous this is. Crawford is especially suspicious of the trend in American labor moving us from the production of goods to the creation of brands. Of all usages of social media this is the most insidious, a noxious concoction of smoke and mirrors that displays aspiration void of integrity. It is also the final merging of personality and capitalism; entrepreneurial "experts" claim that your online persona (and often real-time personality) must be that brand. The bigger problem is the complete disassociation of the mind and body that is a trademark of modern office life. While I could at least walk ten feet to confront my boss, most of us are completely removed from the process of product creation, creating a vast divide between creator and consumer as well as creator and the product created. With no tactile sense of what you're doing, with nothing physical to show for the forty-plus hours a week you spend indoors in anatomically compromised positions staring at a screen under fluorescent lights, it seems impossible to avoid being consumed by an emotional cocoon, one combated with alcohol, opioids, SSRI medication, sleep aids, or, if health is a concern, an hour on a fluorescent that offers little actual divergence from the eight you just spent locked inside another machine.

This is simply not what the human body was designed for. We are adaptable animals, but we cannot keep our bodies locked in passive captivity for large stretches of time and expect to function optimally, nor can we dull our brains with repetitive tasks that require no creative input without losing something essential in our imagination. Contrary to what many believe, our brains are not 'designed' for any specific purpose beyond survival. Evolution does not have big plans in mind; we make it up as this planet moves along. Daniel Levitin puts it best: "There is no overarching grand planner engineering the systems so that they work harmoniously together. The brain is more like a big, old house with piecemeal renovations done on every floor, and less like new construction."[5]

While some find this pessimistic, I argue the reverse. Think of the endless variations of imagination you have the potential to implement every single day. We still have to work with what we have, however, and according to Levitin, we're not doing the best job at it. In 2011, he writes, Americans took in five times the amount of information than twenty-five years prior.[6] That equates to roughly 100,000 words *every day*, and that's only counting leisure time. We might think the information age is a blessing, but we're paying for it, mostly with our attention.

Our brain's processing limit is 120 bits per second. Since having a conversation requires sixty bits, it's hard to respond or make any sense of what the person is saying if you're texting or otherwise distracted. Distraction is the cunning cohort of technology. Websites thrive on it by tempting you with a special offer from a trusted advertiser or by linking to article after article to keep their page counts high, which in turn allows them to sell that trusted space for more money. Social media relies on distraction as well: a fifteen-second Snapchat, a 140-character tweet. When Instagram expanded its video capabilities from fifteen seconds to a minute, it wasn't forcing culture to adapt to longform, it was merely trying to hit the

YouTube viewing sweet spot. That's roughly the limit for most users before they become distracted by another video, Snapchat, or something, anything but what's right in front of them already.

This constant shifting is destroying many neurological capabilities, including emotional regulation and memory. Take multitasking, which is effectively what you're doing while at work logged in to all of your social media accounts and various sundry networks. You might think you're getting more work done, but you're not. What you're doing is elevating levels of cortisol and adrenaline. The dopamine addiction that's created from jumping around exploits your brain's prefrontal cortex, ironically the same place required for attention.[7] Instead of focusing, your fingers anxiously trigger whatever network shows any sign of life, which at this point is all of them. Anxiety created by this constant craving for stimulation increases your body's need for glucose while escalating the likelihood you'll engage in aggressive and impulsive behavior.[8] The result of perpetually seeking novelty, writes physician Siddhartha Mukherjee, is to "try to amplify the signal by stimulating their brains with higher and higher forms of risk. They are like habituated drug users, or like the rats in the dopamine-reward experiment—except the 'drug' is a brain chemical that signals excitement itself."[9]

Human behavior is shaped by dopamine. More than a feel-good neurotransmitter, it influences our actions by ensuring the pleasure we receive from an experience can be replicated later. But remember what happens with music: you receive that dopamine hit *before* the beat drops. The same thing happens when you're hungry. Your brain drips dopamine while seeking nourishment, not when you've actually found it.[10] By gorging on streams of constant entertainment and information, we're never engaging in what Nicolas Carr refers to as "deep thinking."[11] This has detrimental effects, as it reduces our ability to practice empathy and compassion. Instead of displaying concern for others, we stay locked in the glass cage twenty-four inches in front of our downturned faces.

In the fall of 2015 my fiancée scored a pair of tickets to *Real Time with Bill Maher*. If you've never been to a live taping, you have to arrive a few hours early, go through security, and wait. Outside of the studio is a long row of seats for roughly an hour of anticipation. As you head through security before reaching those seats, the staff takes your phones away. What that meant for the few hundred of us gathered on a glorious autumn day in Los Angeles was conversation: everyone was talking to everyone else. No slumped shoulders, no busy eyes, no trigger fingers, and, thank goodness, no selfies. It felt . . . human.

Computers are not dissimilar from rudimentary stone tools our ancestors laboriously carved. They are extensions of our ability to navigate our environment while influencing our behavior. The irony, of course, is that the more advanced we become as toolmakers, they less we are actually able to navigate. To compensate for this loss we rely more and more on external aids. In this process a primal piece of our innate architecture is destroyed. Convenience is not always the key to success; the mismatches our drive toward automation creates are literally and figuratively killing us.

To finish the thought: I'm no Luddite, though in some ways I am. The refusal to be plugged in just because I'm bored; my seemingly counterintuitive decision to not use the vocal commands on GPS so that I'm forced to pay attention to the road (my relationship to space) no matter how often I get lost; my passion for running up and down mountains instead of hopping on a treadmill; choosing to swing a cumbersome kettlebell instead of relying on the smooth trajectory of pulley machines; reading paperbacks instead of screens—these and more are proactive choices I've made to maintain memory, develop emotional regulation, and enhance learning and proprioception skills. This does not mean I don't engage in social media or eschew apps. I simply try my best to keep technology in the basement, where it belongs.

THE SIMPLE TRUTH OF COMPLEXITY

Physical fitness has exploded. Health clubs pull in $75 billion worldwide, counting 131 million members.[12] More than personal development, this drive toward fitness is shaped by community. People like working out together. Instructors enjoy leading others through movement; students love the complexity involved in diverse routines. From CrossFit to yoga, ultramarathons to Tough Mudder races, the knowledge that others are struggling and sweating and growing alongside you is an essential component to physical and emotional health. We're social creatures. Journalist Jason Kelly goes as far to write, "Fitness also has crept into a personal and social space once occupied by organized religion, and it's not just yoga studios and meditation clubs."[13]

Complexity and challenge are key factors in growth. In the follow-up to his bestselling *Flow*, Mihaly Csíkszentmihályi reported on three decades of research regarding the process by which people become creative. While we often associate creativity with innate skills, the psychologist knew it could be developed as a skill and mindset. Making sense of the process of learning how to be creative, he writes, "If I had to express in one word what makes their personalities different from others, it's complexity. They show tendencies of thought and action that in most people are segregated. They contain contradictory extremes; instead of being an individual, each of them is a multitude."[14]

We are more willing to partake in complex workouts when next to others. Of all the anthropology and evolutionary biology cited in this book, this is the most important: humans are tribal animals. We need one another; we rely on each other. When arriving at Equinox or when traveling to workshops and trainings, I get to move with a group of people in ways that collectively make us stronger, more flexible, fitter, and, given what we know about exercise's role in emotional processing, more compassionate and empathic humans. From my years of doing this, this is the best advice I can offer: move often, move in varied ways, and keep moving. You can't stop movement. It's what our bodies do; it's what our brain does. You can control how your body and brain moves, however. The more control you learn, the stronger a body and mind you develop.

This means exercising your brain. While there are many apps that offer "brain training," here are a few strengthening exercises that Philip Steir and I developed to inspire creativity for our Flow Play program at Equinox. They are not puzzles, but rather ways of rethinking your relationship to the world. When teaching yoga I often have my students come into and out of the same poses in novel ways to remind them that there is not one fundamental truth about how the world operates. By changing your perspective on familiar tasks—for example, even trying something as simple as transitioning from Warrior One in a few different ways—you might learn something new along the way. These four exercises are the mental version of that idea:

- Strengthen and prepare your mind by working intensely on a problem, then give yourself a release by doing something completely different. During the break furnish your brain with diverse ideas. Watch a documentary, visit a museum, attend a concert, go for a run somewhere new, or take a scenic drive. Immerse yourself in a novel activity, as it will help your brain discover connections to seemingly spontaneous events. It might even offer you new avenues of thinking about the initial problem.
- Change your perspective on a task; it will help produce novel solutions. Imagine how your parents, best friend, a lawyer, vegan, scientist, terrorist, religious guru, and right wing politician would approach the problem. Alter your frame of reference to see through new eyes. Many of our online interactions are instinctive and reactive and not necessarily well thought out. A common debate tactic is to argue opposing sides of an argument to give you a greater understanding of what's being debated. The next time you find yourself answering with your gut, think it over from the "other side." You may not change your mind, but you may discover something in the process.
- Make analogues by applying the "is like" rule. For example: Attracting more people to my fitness class is like a farmers market vendor trying to get more customers. Sketch the many ways the vendor would go about doing this task. Picking a person completely unrelated to your goal broadens your perspective on how to expand your own pursuits.
- Imagine doing the exact opposite of every solution you have come up with so far and see what creative ideas you come up with.

Look how fitness is usually presented in modern culture: ripped abs, toned arms, flexible spines. Sexiness sells; form is important. Your trainer doesn't have to look like a cover model, but if he moves like a walrus you won't be inspired. You want results, so you need to see how things are properly done. When we look at someone who has obviously put in the time and energy to take care of their bodies we're inspired to do the same. Hopefully through these pages you've realized that what magazine editors choose to put on their covers is a sales technique, not necessarily representative of health. Remember the difference between fitness and health. The two don't always see eye to eye, which is why I'm closing with the most overlooked technique in all of fitness. Strangely, as essential as it is, many pride themselves on *not* doing it, or doing as little as possible, proving how far removed from the natural cycles of life we've become. Still, that one-third of our lives we spend asleep is necessary for healthy bodies and minds. No amount of caffeine we ingest, sprints we run, or time we spend in meditation can erase our need to be unconscious. Sleep is the most important regeneration tool at our disposal. Just as our brain needs a break from technology for space and sanity, our bodies need to be horizontal for at least seven to nine hours a night. To not sleep, often and well, is the most profound deterrent to health imaginable.

It's a Wrap

This book is filled with a variety of exercises and information to help change potentially damaging habits into healthier ones. We *all* have habits—we're just trying to make better ones stick. One of the best that my wife and I have put into practice is leaving our cell phones out of the bedroom. I've certainly been guilty of checking on this or that while winding down, posting something witty, and seeing what's going on right before we shut down. Upon waking up, I've been known to be right back at it. Now I give myself an hour before bed without a screen; upon waking, I make my morning coffee, feed our cats, and sit down near our front balcony with whatever book I'm currently reading. Only after this ritual is complete do I log in to check my email and begin my workday. On early training and teaching days I don't check social media or email until I return home. This might sound insignificant, but in a world in which over half of my income is derived from being plugged in, giving myself this space is essential. As journalist Michael Harris writes regarding the constant need to be on a digital platform, "efficient communication is not the ultimate goal of human experience."[15]

While we can debate what the ultimate goal is, one thing is certain: without a good night's rest you won't achieve much of anything. The reason I keep the phone away from nighttime glances is due to the suppression of melatonin, the hormone that causes drowsiness and regulates sleep cycles.[16] The blue light is not the only problem, however; length of time staring at the device and brightness levels come into play.[17] What you're gazing at is another issue. Playing video games and texting in the hour leading to sleep increases anxiety levels by triggering a release of cortisol, which also disrupts natural sleep cycles.[18] This is also why I don't check first thing upon waking, as a cortisol burst sets into motion a series of crashes throughout the day. This is also why I wake up to ambient classical music instead of that god-awful buzzer. The chemical rush from being jolted out of sleep lasts until the afternoon.[19]

Technology is only one culprit in our cultural battle with insomnia. One Gallup poll reported that 40 percent of Americans do not meet recommended sleep requirements.[20] While we have individual needs, in general seven hours is required for our body to do proper housekeeping. Even just one night of unrest leads to hormonal issues and immune system suppression; issues with memory and cognition, as well as increased inflammation, also result from a sleepless evening.[21] Perhaps the most interesting function of sleep is the activation of what researchers have termed the "glympathic system." While we're asleep, cerebrospinal fluid flushes unwanted toxins from our brain. These include the protein beta-amyloid and synuclein proteins, which play roles in Alzheimer's, Parkinson's, and multisystem atrophy.[22] Think about what happens to gutters if they're not cleaned after the autumn foliage drops. Staying awake for long stretches is not a badge of honor. It's a toxic build-up of dangerous proteins.

We know lack of sleep as an issue. We have to, since our body will shut down if we avoid it. A bigger problem exists in our most popular solution. In the stretch from 1994 to 2007, prescriptions for nonbenzodiazepine sedative-hypnotics such as zolpidem—Ambien leads the charge—increased over thirty times.[23] This is rather disturbing given the fact that insomnia rates grew only six times during that same period. This pill-for-everything mentality has led to innumerable addictions and deaths with pain relief in the form of opioid abuse. Likewise, sleeping pills do not address the underlying causes of insomnia. They merely add between *eleven and nineteen minutes* of sleep each night.[24] That's right: in exchange for a psychologically addictive pharmaceutical laden with potential side effects, including increased risk of suicide, dizziness, light-headedness, headache, nausea, upset stomach, and feeling tired—the very thing the pill is designed to fix—you're not even getting a sitcom's worth of sleep. At the moment somewhere around seventy million Americans report not sleeping enough, which has resulted in fifty-five million prescriptions topping $1 billion in revenue in 2014 alone.[25] A lack of sleep is also implicated in anxiety and climbing obesity rates, two of the main problems we've discussed. Who'd have thought that we'd come this far only to find out the most important practice we can implement for a healthy lifestyle is the very thing our parents were always telling us to do more of?

It's not that simple, of course. In these pages we've discussed many mismatches we partake in without recognizing the folly in them. Recall that this book is not a definitive outline but a program that requires personal experimentation. That's tough to come to terms with in a culture that's accustomed to being told that this or that change will instantly change their lives. Once the novelty of a solution wears off we're left craving more of that new sensation. The tragedy is in the craving. Health is a slow and thoughtful journey, a lifelong process. It evolves as your body ages. There is no other way of treating it, and that's okay. In fact it's quite beautiful, even poetic.

My forty-two-year-old body is incapable of accomplishing what my eighteen-year-old body did. In its place is something wiser and more mature. During my freshman year at Rutgers my fitness goals involved dunking a basketball and benching above my body weight. Today it's feeling good when I get out of bed in the morning. Sure, my day is filled with students and clients, research and writing, and I have not let go of certain goals in my exercise routines. But those are part of the journey. If there is any goal it's to be pain-free from waking to shut-eye.

The cascade of hormones and neurotransmitters that floods your brain and body before, during, and after cardiovascular exercise is different from the cocktail you receive during yoga, meditation, and sleep. All are essential to your well-being. If you are on the sluggish side, a pick-me-up might be required, or perhaps a scan of your refrigerator to remove what's slowing you down. Being hyper and overexcited has another prescription. My friend and colleague Tommy Rosen, an addiction recovery facilitator, calls his Kundalini yoga workshops "The Infinite Pharmacy Within." While there are many illnesses and diseases that require pharmaceutical interventions, many problems are solvable by a sober and honest investigation of lifestyle choices. Joseph Campbell once remarked, "I don't believe people are looking for the meaning of life as much as they are looking for the experience of being alive."[26] What we're seeking, I surmise, is the sensation of being whole. Funny thing is, we already are. We just need to remove the obscurations and move, think, and feel in ways that remind us being alive is a blessing unto itself.

Acknowledgments

While writing is often portrayed as a solitary affair, it is very much a public discipline, especially a book like this. The thousands of people I have interacted with over my two decades practicing and working in yoga and fitness have influenced what lives and breathes inside of these pages. Many people will be overlooked and for that I apologize. I will keep it to only those that directly influenced the process of producing *Whole Motion*.

The seed of this book was planted when creating Flow Play alongside Philip Steir for Equinox. His valuable insights and research into music's neurological effects led me to pursue many other avenues of neuroscience and psychology, but the entire process began with him. Plus we had a great time traveling the country, nerding out, and flowing.

That program began thanks to Lashaun Dale, an incredible mentor as well as the person who took a chance when hiring me at Equinox in 2004. You never know how a simple decision will end up. Thanks to her I've carved an unforeseeable path in yoga and fitness. Thanks to Lisa Wheeler for helping craft the program as well, and the press and marketing team at Equinox for shining a light on it.

There have been so many instructors who have inspired the work in these pages. I would never have taken movement seriously if not for Brendan McCall, my first dance and yoga teacher, and his unmatched ability to invite students to open up to exploration. To this day I remain influenced by those early Saturday morning hours at NYU. Marc Coronel has been a longtime colleague off of whom I get to bounce ideas, victories, and frustrations in this industry. I know few men with such integrity for movement and science. Plus, we always have a great time chatting and hanging. This book would have been impossible without Amber McMahon, who inspired me to teach main studio and studio cycling. As my manager and mentor she's offered a number of opportunities to a tall, lumbering, wiseass yogi. I greatly appreciate her faith in my evolving journey.

Thanks to my agent, Helen Zimmerman, for taking a different sort of chance on a writer who blindly reached out to her one spring day. Like any relationship, that between a writer and agent is tricky. From the first moment I pitched this idea she understood and embraced it, offering valuable guidance that landed me this book deal. Thanks as well to Skyhorse Publishing for including me in their vast and diverse catalog.

Daniel Housman helped me greatly by offering his eagle eyes and insights as I developed this work. Josh Nelson took all the photographs in these pages. Besides being great with the camera, he's a solid friend. Orion Jones, my editor at Big Think, gave me the space to cover a number of these topics in my column for the site, which I am indebted to. And while he has not seen much of this book, Dax-Devlon Ross and I have spent many hours hiking and discussing the topics. More than theory, he embodies the discipline to take care of himself like few people I've ever met. I'm thankful we've gotten to push one another for over two decades now, on the trail, on the court, and in life.

This book is dedicated to my father, Ferenc, who I talk about in these pages. He's been in great shape his entire life, teaching me why it's so important even when I didn't realize it: picking me up and dropping me off at practices and games, always cheering from the bleachers, teaching me how to field, shooting hoops in our sloping driveway, and inadvertently proving to me that whipping your pitching wedge into a lake after a mis-hit is not the best course of action. We are all works in progress. I am eternally grateful.

While writing is in many ways public, countless hours are spent thinking, researching, struggling, and actually writing. My wife, Callan, has been supportive and enthusiastic throughout this entire process. This is a book about making yourself whole, but there's nothing better than finding someone who helps you accomplish just that.

Notes

Chapter 1

1. Ratey, John J. and Eric Hagerman. *Spark: The Revolutionary New Science of Exercise and the Brain*. New York: Little, Brown, 2008, 2.
2. Llinás, Rodolfo R. *I of the Vortex: From Neurons to Self*. Cambridge: MIT Press, 2001, 5.
3. James, William. *The Principles of Psychology, Vol. 1*. New York: Dover Publications, 1950.

Chapter 2

1. Jaak Panksepp. *The Archaeology of Mind: Neuroevolutionary Origins of Human Emotions*. New York: W. W. Norton and Company, 2012, 95.
2. Metzinger, Thomas. *The Ego Tunnel: The Science of the Mind and the Myth of the Self*. New York: Basic Books, 2009, 15.
3. Gottschall, Jonathan. *The Storytelling Animal: How Stories Make Us Human*. Boston: Houghton Mifflin Harcourt, 2012, loc 237.
4. Kellogg, Ronald Thomas. *The Making of the Mind: The Neuroscience of Human Nature*. Amherst: Prometheus Books, 2013, 51.
5. Bloom, Paul. "Is God an Accident?" *The Atlantic*, December 2005. http://www.theatlantic.com/magazine/archive/2005/12/is-god-an-accident/304425/.
6. Gerstacker, Diana. "Sitting is the New Smoking." *The Huffington Post*, November 26, 2014. http://www.huffingtonpost.com/the-active-times/sitting-is-the-new-smokin_b_5890006.html.

7. Gross, Terry. NPR Fresh Air Tumblr, September 20, 2011. http://nprfreshair.tumblr.com/post/11699441962/memory-is-a-poet-not-an-historian-on-todays.

8. Hurd, Michael D. "The Cost of Dementia: Who Will Pay?" Rand Corporation, May 1, 2013. http://www.rand.org/blog/2013/05/the-cost-of-dementia-who-will-pay.html.

9. Ratey, John J., and Richard Manning. *Go Wild: Eat Fat, Run Free, Be Social, and Follow Evolution's Other Rules for Total Health and Well-being.* New York: Little, Brown, 2015, 107.

10. Ratey, John J., and Eric Hagerman. *Spark: The Revolutionary New Science of Exercise and the Brain.* New York: Little, Brown, 2008, 42.

11. McGonigal, Kelly. *The Upside of Stress: Why Stress Is Good for You, and How to Get Good at It.* New York: Penguin, 2015, 12.

Chapter 3

1. Kolk, Bessel Van Der. *The Body Keeps the Score: Brain, Mind, and Body in the Healing of Trauma.* New York: Penguin, 2015, 79.

2. McGonigal, Kelly. *The Upside of Stress: Why Stress Is Good for You, and How to Get Good at It.* New York: Penguin, 2016, 63–4.

3. McGonigal, Kelly. *The Upside of Stress: Why Stress Is Good for You, and How to Get Good at It.* New York: Penguin, 2016, 50.

4. Kolk, Bessel Van Der. *The Body Keeps the Score: Brain, Mind, and Body in the Healing of Trauma.* New York: Penguin, 2015, 11.

5. Stossel, Scott. *My Age of Anxiety: Fear, Hope, Dread, and the Search for Peace of Mind.* New York: Vintage Books, 2013, 8.

6. LeDoux, Joseph E. *Anxious: Using the Brain to Understand and Treat Fear and Anxiety.* New York: Viking, 2015, 14.

7. LeDoux, Joseph E. *Anxious: Using the Brain to Understand and Treat Fear and Anxiety.* New York: Viking, 2015, 42.

8. "Gauging the Impact of Noise on Children's Learning," *Metrofocus*, August 28, 2012. http://www.thirteen.org/metrofocus/2012/08/gauging-the-impact-of-noise-on-childrens-learning/

9. Krause, Bernard L. *The Great Animal Orchestra: Finding the Origins of Music in the World's Wild Places*. New York: Little, Brown, 2012, 164.

10. Neilson, Susie. "Noise Is a Drug and New York Is Full of Addicts." *Nautilus*, July 2016, 70–79.

11. McGonigal, Kelly. *The Upside of Stress: Why Stress Is Good for You, and How to Get Good at It*. New York: Penguin, 2016, 66.

12. Miller, Jill. *The Roll Model: A Step-by-step Guide to Erase Pain, Improve Mobility, and Live Better in Your Body*. Las Vegas: Victory Belt Publishing, 2014, 97.

13. Miller, Jill. *The Roll Model: A Step-by-step Guide to Erase Pain, Improve Mobility, and Live Better in Your Body*. Las Vegas: Victory Belt Publishing, 2014, 104.

Chapter 4

1. Fortey, Richard A. *Life: A Natural History of the First Four Billion Years of Life on Earth*. New York, NY: Alfred A. Knopf, 1998, 40.

2. Dennett, Daniel C. *From Bacteria to Bach and Back: The Evolution of Minds*. New York: W. W. Norton & Company, 2017, 8.

3. Stossel, Scott. *My Age of Anxiety: Fear, Hope, Dread, and the Search for Peace of Mind*. New York: Vintage Books, 2013, 8.

4. LeDoux, Joseph E. *Anxious: Using the Brain to Understand and Treat Fear and Anxiety*. New York: Viking, 2015, 43.

5. Harari, Yuval N. *Sapiens: A Brief History of Humankind*. New York: HarperCollins Publishers, 2015, 8.

6. Zemach-Bersin, David. "The Feldenkrais Method, 'Better Turning,' Part One of an Awareness Through Movement Lesson." https://www.youtube.com/watch?v=ZSletIPIN30.

7. Doidge, Norman. *The Brain's Way of Healing: Remarkable Discoveries and Recoveries from the Frontiers of Neuroplasticity*. New York: Penguin, 2015, 165.

8. Griffiths, Sarah. "The exercise that predicts your DEATH: Struggling with 'sitting-rising test' means you're 5 times more

likely to die early." *Daily Mail*, December 3, 2016. http://www.dailymail.co.uk/sciencetech/article-2858804/Can-exercise-test-predict-DEATH-People-struggle-sitting-rising-test-five-times-likely-die.html.

9. Feldenkrais, Moshé. *Awareness Through Movement: Easy-to-do Exercises to Improve Your Posture, Vision, Imagination, and Personal Awareness.* New York: HarperOne, 2009, 36.

10. Sihvonen, R., M. Paavola, A. Itälä, A. Joukainen, J. Kalske, T. L. Järvinen. "Arthroscopic Partial Meniscectomy versus Sham Surgery for a Degenerative Meniscal Tear." *The New England Journal of Medicine* (December 26, 2013): 2515-2524. http://www.nejm.org/doi/full/10.1056/NEJMoa1305189

11. Alfini, A. J., L. R. Weisee, B. P. Leitner, T. J. Smith, J. M. Hagberg, J. Smith Carson. "Hippocampal and Cerebral Blood Flow after Exercise Cessation in Master Athletes." *Frontiers in Aging Neuroscience* (August 5, 2016).

12. McGreevey, Sue. "Eight weeks to a better brain." *Harvard Gazette*, January 21, 2011. http://news.harvard.edu/gazette/story/2011/01/eight-weeks-to-a-better-brain/.

Chapter 5

1. McDougall, Christopher. *Born to Run: A Hidden Tribe, Super-athletes, and the Greatest Race the World Has Never Seen.* New York: Vintage, 2011, 221.

2. Van Gent, R. N. "Incidence and determinants of lower extremity running injuries in long distance runners: a systematic review." *British Journal of Sports Medicine* (March 12, 2007).

3. "Athletic Footwear Market to Value USD 84.4 billion by 2018, Could Grow at CAGR of 1.8% From 2012–2018: Transparency Market Research." PR Newswire, July 9, 2015. http://www.prnewswire.com/news-releases/athletic-footwear-market-to-value-usd-844-billion-by-2018-could-grow-at-cagr-of-18-from-2012—2018-transparency-market-research-512842661.html.

4. Fishman, Loren, and Ellen Saltonstall. *Yoga for Osteoporosis.* New York: W. W. Norton & Company, 2010, 5.
5. Boman, Katy. *Whole Body Barefoot: Transitioning to Minimal Footwear.* Sequim: Propriometrics Press, 2015, 11.
6. Lieberman, Daniel. *The Story of the Human Body: Evolution, Health, and Disease.* New York City, NY: Vintage Books, 2014, 326.
7. Murakami, Haruki. *What I Talk About When I Talk About Running.* New York: Vintage, 2009, 20.
8. Laursen, Paul B., and David G. Jenkins. "The Scientific Basis for High-Intensity Interval Training." School of Human Movement Studies. http://www.tradewindsports.net/wp-content/uploads/2013/10/Laursen-02-Scien-Basis-for-HIIT-Review.pdf.
9. Chapman, Sandra B., Sina Aslan, Jeffrey S. Spence, Laura F. DeFina, Molly W. Keebler, Nyaz Dibehbani, and Hanzhang Lu. "Shorter term aerobic exercise improves brain, cognition, and cardiovascular fitness in aging." *Frontiers in Aging Neuroscience* (November 12, 2013). http://journal.frontiersin.org/article/10.3389/fnagi.2013.00075/full.

Chapter 6

1. Archibald, Dresdin. "The History of Weight Sports: How They Evolved Since 1900." *Breaking Muscle.* http://breakingmuscle.com/olympic-weightlifting/the-history-of-weight-sports-how-they-evolved-since-1900.
2. Reynolds, Gretchen. "Phys Ed: Brains and Brawn." *New York Times,* January 19, 2011. http://well.blogs.nytimes.com/2011/01/19/phys-ed-brains-and-brawn/?_r=1.
3. Yarrow, Joshua F., Lesley J. White, Sean C. McCoy, and Stephen E. Borst. "Training Augments Resistance Exercise Induced Elevation of Circulating Brain Derived Neurotrophic Factor (BDNF)." *Neuroscience Letters* 479, no. 2 (2010): 161–65.
4. Bolandzadeh, N., R. Tam, T. C. Handy, L. S. Nagamatsu, J. C. Davis, E. Dao, B. L. Beattie, and T. Liu-Ambrose. "Resistance Training and White Matter Lesion Progression in Older

Women: Exploratory Analysis of a 12-Month Randomized Controlled Trial." *Journal of American Geriatric Society* (October 2015). http://www.ncbi.nlm.nih.gov/pubmed/26456233.

5. Weinberg, Lisa, Anita Hasni, Minoru Shinohara, and Audry Duarte. "A single bout of resistance exercise can enhance episodic memory performance." *Acta Psychologica* (November 2014): 13–19. http://www.sciencedirect.com/science/article/pii/S0001691814001577.

6. "Build Muscle Without External Load?" *IDEA Fitness Journal,* September 2016, 12.

7. Duvall, Jeremy. "Trainer Q&A: Should I Always Lift Weights to Failure?" *Men's Fitness.* http://www.mensfitness.com/training/pro-tips/trainer-qa-should-i-always-lift-weights-failure.

8. Harford, Tim. *Adapt: Why Success Always Starts with Failure.* New York: Farrar, Straus and Giroux, 2011, 224.

9. Dweck, Carol S. *Mindset: The New Psychology of Success.* New York: Random House, 2006, 99–100.

10. Dweck, Carol S. "Caution-Praise Can Be Dangerous." *American Educator,* Spring 1999.

11. Dweck, Carol S. "Caution-Praise Can Be Dangerous." *American Educator,* Spring 1999.

Chapter 7

1. Varenne, Jean. *Yoga and the Hindu Tradition.* Chicago: University of Chicago Press, 1976, 1.

2. White, David Gordon. *The Yoga Sutra of Patanjali: A Biography.* Princeton: Princeton University Press, 2014.

3. Eliade, Mircea. *Yoga: Immortality and Freedom.* Princeton: Princeton University Press, 1990, xvii.

4. Singleton, Mark. *Yoga Body: The Origins of Modern Posture Practice.* Oxford: Oxford University Press, 2010.

5. "2016 Yoga in America Study Conducted by Yoga Journal & Yoga Alliance." 2016 Yoga in America Study. January 13, 2016. https://www.yogaalliance.org/2016yogainamericastudy.

6. Chui, D.H., M. Marcellino, F. Marotta, H. Sweed, A. I. Vigali, W. Xiao, A. Ayala, U. Cagnuolo, and N. Zerbinati. "A double-blind, rct testing beneficial modulation of BDNF in middle-aged, life style-stressed subjects: a clue to brain protection?" *Journal of Clinical and Diagnostic Research* (November 20, 2014). http://www.ncbi.nlm.nih.gov/pubmed/25584253.
7. Broad, William J. *The Science of Yoga: The Risks and the Rewards*. New York, NY: Simon & Schuster, 2012, 100.
8. Streeter, Chris C. "Effects of Yoga Versus Walking on Mood, Anxiety, and Brain GABA Levels: A Randomized Controlled MRS Study." *Journal of Alternative and Complementary Medicine* (November 2010).
9. Korb, Alex. "Yoga: Changing the Brain's Stressful Habits." *Psychology Today*, September 7, 2011. https://www.psychologytoday.com/blog/prefrontal-nudity/201109/yoga-changing-the-brains-stressful-habits.
10. Beres, Derek. *The Warrior's Path: Living Yoga's Ten Codes*. Los Angeles: Outside the Box Publishing, 2014.

Chapter 8

1. Thompson, Evan. *Waking, Dreaming, Being: Self and Consciousness in Neuroscience, Meditation, and Philosophy*. New York: Columbia University Press, 2014.
2. Zeidan, Fadel, Susan K. Johnson, Bruce J. Diamond, Zhanna David, and Paula Goolkasian. "Mindfulness meditation improves cognition: Evidence of brief mental training." *Consciousness and Cognition*, Volume 19, Issue 2 (June 2010): 597–605.
3. Carlson, L.E., and S. N. Garland. "Impact of mindfulness-based stress reduction (MBSR) on sleep, mood, stress and fatigue symptoms in cancer outpatients." *International Journal of Behavioral Medicine* (2005): 278–85.
4. Price, C. J., B. McBride, L. Hyerle, and D. R. Kivlahan. "Mindful awareness in bodyoriented therapy for female veterans with post-traumatic stress disorder taking prescription

analgesics for chronic pain: a feasibility study." *Alternative Therapies in Health and Medicine* (2007): 32–40.

5. Lazar, S. W., G. Bush, R. L. Gollub, G. L. Fricchione, G. Khalsa, and H. Benson. "Functional brain mapping of the relaxation response and meditation." *Neuroreport* (May 15 2000): 1581–1585.

6. Travis, F, Shear, J. "Focused attention, open monitoring and automatic self-transcending: Categories to organize meditations from Vedic, Buddhist and Chinese traditions." *Consciousness and Cognition*, Vol. 19, Issue 4 (December 2010): 1110–1118.

7. Davidson, Richard J. *The Emotional Life of Your Brain*. London: Plume, 2012, 113.

8. Davidson, Richard J. *The Emotional Life of Your Brain*. London: Plume, 2012, 125.

9. Davidson, Richard J. *The Emotional Life of Your Brain*. London: Plume, 2012, 155.

10. Davidson, Richard J. *The Emotional Life of Your Brain*. London: Plume, 2012, 210.

11. Kellogg, Ronald Thomas. *The Making of the Mind: The Neuroscience of Human Nature*. Amherst: Prometheus Books, 2013, 40.

12. Kellogg, Ronald Thomas. *The Making of the Mind: The Neuroscience of Human Nature*. Amherst: Prometheus Books, 2013, 22.

13. Feuerstein, Georg. *The Yoga-Sutra of Patanjali*. Rochester: Inner Traditions International, 1989, 26.

14. Damasio, Antonio. *Self Comes to Mind*. New York: Vintage, 2010, loc. 201.

15. Payne, Jessica D., and Lynn Nadel. "Sleep, dreams, and memory consolidation: The role of the stress hormone cortisol." Learning & Memory (2004): 671–678. http://learnmem.cshlp .org/content/11/6/671.full

16. Harris, Sam. *Waking Up: A Guide to Spirituality Without Religion*. New York: Simon & Schuster, 2014, 101.

17. Levitin, Dan. *The Organized Mind: Thinking Straight in the Age of Information Overload*. New York: Dutton, 2014, 45.

18. Metzinger, Thomas. *The Ego Tunnel: The Science of the Mind and the Myth of the Self.* New York: Basic Books, 2009, 7.
19. Metzinger, Thomas. *The Ego Tunnel: The Science of the Mind and the Myth of the Self.* New York: Basic Books, 2009, 9.
20. Harris, Sam. *Waking Up: A Guide to Spirituality Without Religion.* New York: Simon & Schuster, 2014, 35.
21. Davidson, Richard J. *The Emotional Life of Your Brain.* London: Plume, 2012, 242.

Chapter 9

1. Duhigg, Charles. *The Power of Habit: Why We Do What We Do in Life and Business.* New York: Random House, 2012.
2. DiSalvo, David. "What Alcohol Really Does to Your Brain." *Forbes,* October 16, 2012. http://www.forbes.com/sites/daviddisalvo/2012/10/16/what-alcohol-really-does-to-your-brain/#22925ea2413b.
3. Wright, Robert. *The Moral Animal: The New Science of Evolutionary Psychology.* New York: Pantheon Books, 1994, 186.
4. Lieberman, Daniel. *The Story of the Human Body: Evolution, Health, and Disease.* New York: Vintage, 2014, 54.

Chapter 10

1. Tudge, Colin. *Neanderthals, Bandits & Farmers: How Agriculture Really Began.* New Haven: Yale University Press, 1999, 3.
2. Junger, Sebastian. *Tribe: On Homecoming and Belonging.* New York: Twelve, 2016, 17.
3. Lieberman, Daniel. *The Story of the Human Body: Evolution, Health, and Disease.* New York: Vintage Books, 2014, 173.
4. Mithen, Stephen. *The Prehistory of the Mind: The Cognitive Origins of Art, Religion and Science.* London: Thames and Hudson, 1996, 218–9.
5. Ratey, John J., and Richard Manning. *Go Wild: Eat Fat, Run Free, Be Social, and Follow Evolution's Other Rules for Total Health and Well-being.* New York: Little, Brown, 2015, 92.

6. "Adult Obesity Causes & Consequences." Center for Disease Control and Prevention. https://www.cdc.gov/obesity/adult/causes.html

7. "The Strange History of Frozen Food: From Clarence Birdseye to the Distinguished Order of Zerocrats." *Eater*, August 21, 2014. http://www.eater.com/2014/8/21/6214423/the-strange-history-of-frozen-food-from-clarence-birdseye-to-the

8. Hazell, Krysty. "Fatty and Sugary Foods Are As Addictive As Cocaine And Nicotine, Warn Health Experts." *Huffington Post UK*, January 3, 2012. http://www.huffingtonpost.co.uk/2011/11/03/fatty-and-sugary-food-as-addictive-as-cocaine-and-nicotine_n_1073513.html

9. Mukherjee, Siddhartha. *The Gene: An Intimate History*. New York, NY: Scribner, 2016, 264.

10. Hyman, Mark. *Eat Fat, Get Thin: Why the Fat We Eat Is the Key to Sustained Weight Loss and Vibrant Health*. New York: Little, Brown and Company, 2016, 13.

11. Hyman, Mark. *Eat Fat, Get Thin: Why the Fat We Eat Is the Key to Sustained Weight Loss and Vibrant Health*. New York: Little, Brown and Company, 2016, 33.

12. Lieberman, Daniel. *The Story of the Human Body: Evolution, Health, and Disease*. New York: Vintage Books, 2014, 117.

13. Hyman, Mark. *Eat Fat, Get Thin: Why the Fat We Eat Is the Key to Sustained Weight Loss and Vibrant Health*. New York: Little, Brown and Company, 2016, 27.

14. Kolata, Gina. "After 'The Biggest Loser,' Their Bodies Fought to Regain Weight." *New York Times*, May 2, 2016. http://www.nytimes.com/2016/05/02/health/biggest-loser-weight-loss.html

15. Belluz, Julia, and Javier Zarracina. "Why you shouldn't exercise to lose weight, explained with 60+ studies." *Vox*, April 28, 2016. http://www.vox.com/2016/4/28/11518804/weight-loss-exercise-myth-burn-calories

16. Ratey, John J., and Richard Manning. *Go Wild: Eat Fat, Run Free, Be Social, and Follow Evolution's Other Rules for Total Health and Well-being*. New York: Little, Brown, 2015, 85.

17. Hyman, Mark. *Eat Fat, Get Thin: Why the Fat We Eat Is the Key to Sustained Weight Loss and Vibrant Health.* New York: Little, Brown and Company, 2016, 74.
18. Lieberman, Daniel. *The Story of the Human Body: Evolution, Health, and Disease.* New York: Vintage Books, 2014, 282.
19. Pollan, Michael. *Cooked: A Natural History of Transformation.* New York: Penguin, 2014, 3.
20. Whybrow, Peter C. *The Well-Tuned Brain: The Remedy for a Manic Society.* New York: W. W. Norton & Compnay, 2015, 39.
21. Pollan, Michael. *Cooked: A Natural History of Transformation.* New York: Penguin, 2014, 229.

Chapter 11

1. Csíkszentmihályi, Mihaly. *Flow: The Psychology of Optimal Experience.* New York: Harper & Row, 1990, 2.
2. Kotler, Steven. "Flow States and Creativity." *Psychology Today,* February 25, 2014. https://www.psychologytoday.com/blog/the-playing-field/201402/flow-states-and-creativity.
3. Batuman, Elif. "Electrified." *The New Yorker,* March 30, 2015. http://www.newyorker.com/magazine/2015/04/06/electrified.
4. Hill, Patrick. "Having a Sense of Purpose May Add Years to Your Life." *Association for Psychological Science,* May 12, 2014. http://www.psychologicalscience.org/news/releases/having-a-sense-of-purpose-in-life-may-add-years-to-your-life.html#.WCZKlZMrJTY
5. Csíkszentmihályi, Mihaly. *Flow: The Psychology of Optimal Experience.* New York: Harper & Row, 1990, 7.
6. Frankl, Viktor E. *Man's Search for Meaning.* Boston: Beacon Press, 2006.
7. Campbell, Joseph, Phil Cousineau, and Stuart L. Brown. *The Hero's Journey: The World of Joseph Campbell: Joseph Campbell on His Life and Work.* San Francisco: Harper & Row, 1990, 217.
8. Clark, Carla. "Can You Improve Physical Skills While Dreaming?" *BrainBlogger,* Sept 8, 2016. http://brainblogger.com/

2016/09/08/can-you-improve-physical-skills-while-dreaming/

9. McDougall, Christopher. *Born to Run: A Hidden Tribe, Super-athletes, and the Greatest Race the World Has Never Seen.* New York, NY: Vintage Books, 2009, 94.

Chapter 12

1. Gottschall, Jonathan. *The Storytelling Animal: How Stories Make Us Human.* Boston: Houghton Mifflin Harcourt, 2012.

2. Baker, Mitzi. "Music Moves Brain to Pay Attention, Stanford Study Finds." News Center, August 1, 2007. https://med.stanford.edu/news/all-news/2007/07/music-moves-brain-to-pay-attention-stanford-study-finds.html.

3. Padnani, Amisha. "The Power of Music, Tapped in a Cubicle." *New York Times*, August 11, 2012. http://www.nytimes.com/2012/08/12/jobs/how-music-can-improve-worker-productivity-workstation.html?_r=0.

4. Vijayalakshmi, K., Susmita Sridhar, and Payal Khanwani. "Estimation of Effects of Alpha Music on EEG Components by Time and Frequency Domain Analysis." International Conference on Computer and Communication Engineering (ICCCE'10) (2010).

5. Yong, Ed. "The dark side of oxytocin, much more than just a 'love hormone.'" *Discover*, November 29, 2010. http://blogs.discovermagazine.com/notrocketscience/2010/11/29/the-dark-side-of-oxytocin-much-more-than-just-a-love-hormone/#.V8yzvZMrJTY.

6. "Imperfect Harmony: How Singing With Others Changes Your Life." NPR, June 3, 2013. http://www.npr.org/2013/06/03/188355968/imperfect-harmony-how-chorale-singing-changes-lives.

7. Storr, Anthony. *Music and the Mind.* New York: Free Press, 1992.

8. Nilsson, Ulrica. "Soothing Music Can Increase Oxytocin Levels during Bed Rest after Open-heart Surgery: A Randomised

Control Trial." *Journal of Clinical Nursing* 18, no. 15 (2009): 2153-161.

9. Moisse, Katie, and ABC News Medical Unit. "Music Therapy Helps Gabrielle Giffords Find Her Voice After Tucson Shooting." *ABC News*, March 08, 2011. http://abcnews.go.com/Health/Wellness/gabrielle-giffords-music-therapy-rewires-brain-tragedy-tucson/story?id= 13075593.

10. Pacchetti, Claudio, Francesca Mancini, Roberto Aglieri, Cira Fundarò, Emilia Martignoni, and Giuseppe Nappi. "Active Music Therapy in Parkinson's Disease: An Integrative Method for Motor and Emotional Rehabilitation." *Psychosomatic Medicine* 62, no. 3 (2000): 386–93.

11. Levitin, Daniel J. *The World in Six Songs: How the Musical Brain Created Human Nature.* New York: Dutton, 2008.

12. Krause, Bernard L. *The Great Animal Orchestra: Finding the Origins of Music in the World's Wild Places*, pp 162–4. New York: Little, Brown, 2012.

Chapter 13

1. Carr, Nicholas. *The Glass Cage: How Our Computers Are Changing Us.* New York, NY: W.W. Norton & Company, 2014, 67.

2. Carr, Nicholas. *The Glass Cage: How Our Computers Are Changing Us.* New York, NY: W.W. Norton & Company, 2014, 73.

3. Carr, Nicholas. *The Glass Cage: How Our Computers Are Changing Us.* New York, NY: W.W. Norton & Company, 2014, 84.

4. Crawford, Matthew B. *Shop Class as Soul Craft: An Inquiry Into the Value of Work.* London: Penguin, 2010, 56.

5. Levitin, Daniel J. *The Organized Mind: Thinking Straight in the Age of Information Overload.* New York, NY: Dutton, 2014, xix.

6. Levitin, Daniel J. *The Organized Mind: Thinking Straight in the Age of Information Overload.* New York, NY: Dutton, 2014, 6.

7. Levitin, Daniel J. *The Organized Mind: Thinking Straight in the Age of Information Overload.* New York, NY: Dutton, 2014, 96.

8. Levitin, Daniel J. *The Organized Mind: Thinking Straight in the Age of Information Overload.* New York, NY: Dutton, 2014, 98.

9. Mukherjee, Siddhartha. *The Gene: An Intimate History.* New York, NY: Scribner, 2016, 386.

10. LeDoux, Joseph E. *Anxious: Using the Brain to Understand and Treat Fear and Anxiety.* New York, NY: Viking, 2015, 142.

11. Carr, Nicholas G. *The Shallows: What the Internet Is Doing to Our Brains.* New York: W.W. Norton, 2010, 216.

12. Kelly, Jason. *Sweat Equity: Inside the New Economy of Mind and Body.* Hoboken, NJ: John Wiley & Sons, 2016, 35.

13. Kelly, Jason. *Sweat Equity: Inside the New Economy of Mind and Body.* Hoboken, NJ: John Wiley & Sons, 2016, 28.

14. Csikszentmihalyi, Mihaly. *Creativity: The Psychology of Discovery and Invention.* New York: Harper Collins Publishers, 2013.

15. Harris, Michael. *The End of Absence: Reclaiming What We've Lost in a World of Constant Connection.* New York, NY: Current, 2015, 71.

16. Cajochen, C., S. Frey, D. Anders, J. Spati, M. Bues, A. Pross, R. Mager, A. Wirz-Justice, and O. Stefani. "Evening Exposure to a Light-emitting Diodes (LED)-backlit Computer Screen Affects Circadian Physiology and Cognitive Performance." *Journal of Applied Physiology* 110, no. 5 (2011): 1432–438.

17. Wood, Brittany, Mark S. Rea, Barbara Plitnick, and Mariana G. Figueiro. "Light Level and Duration of Exposure Determine the Impact of Self-luminous Tablets on Melatonin Suppression." *Applied Ergonomics* 44, no. 2 (2013): 237–40.

18. Rettner, Rachael. "Nighttime Gadget Use Interferes with Young Adults' Health." *Live Science,* March 10, 2011. http://www.livescience.com/35536-technology-sleep-adolescents.html.

19. Campbell, Don, and Alex Doman. *Healing at the Speed of Sound: How What We Hear Transforms Our Brains and Our Lives.* New York: Plume, 2012.

20. Jones, Jeffrey M. "In U.S., 40% Get Less Than Recommended Amount of Sleep." Gallup.com. December 19, 2013. http://

www.gallup.com/poll/166553/less-recommended-amount-sleep.aspx.

21. Stickgold, Robert. "Sleep On It!" *Scientific American*, October 2015, 52–57.

22. Nedergaard, Maiken, and Steven A. Goldman. "Brain Drain." *Scientific American*, March 2016, 45–49.

23. Romm, Cari. "Americans Are Getting Worse at Taking Sleeping Pills." *The Atlantic*, August 12, 2014. http://www.theatlantic.com/health/archive/2014/08/americans-are-getting-worse-at-taking-sleeping-pills/375935/.

24. Saul, Stephanie. "Sleep Drugs Found Only Mildly Effective, but Wildly Popular." *New York Times*, October 23, 2007. http://www.nytimes.com/2007/10/23/health/23drug.html.

25. Huffington, Arianna. *The Sleep Revolution: Transforming Your Life, One Night at a Time*. New York: Harmony Books, 2016, 47.

26. Campbell, Joseph, and Diane K. Osbon (editor). *A Joseph Campbell Companion: Reflections on the Art of Living*. New York: Harper Perennial, 1995.